THE MICROBIOME
WHAT EVERYONE NEEDS TO KNOW®

THE MICROBIOME
WHAT EVERYONE NEEDS TO KNOW®

BERENICE LANGDON

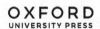

OXFORD
UNIVERSITY PRESS

Oxford University Press is a department of the University of Oxford.
It furthers the University's objective of excellence in research, scholarship,
and education by publishing worldwide. Oxford is a registered trade mark of
Oxford University Press in the UK and in certain other countries.

"What Everyone Needs to Know" is a registered trademark
of Oxford University Press.

Published in the United States of America by Oxford University Press
198 Madison Avenue, New York, NY 10016, United States of America.

© Oxford University Press 2025

All rights reserved. No part of this publication may be reproduced, stored in a retrieval system,
transmitted, used for text and data mining, or used for training artificial intelligence, in any form or
by any means, without the prior permission in writing of Oxford University Press, or as expressly
permitted by law, by license or under terms agreed with the appropriate reprographics rights
organization. Inquiries concerning reproduction outside the scope of the above should be sent
to the Rights Department, Oxford University Press, at the address above.

You must not circulate this work in any other form
and you must impose this same condition on any acquirer.

CIP data is on file at the Library of Congress

ISBN 9780197695609
ISBN 9780197695593 (hbk.)

DOI: 10.1093/WENTK/9780197695593.001.0001

Paperback printed by Integrated Books International, United States of America
Hardback printed by Lightning Source, Inc., United States of America

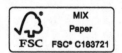

The manufacturer's authorised representative in the EU for product safety is Oxford
University Press España S.A., Parque Empresarial San Fernando de Henares,
Avenida de Castilla, 2 – 28830 Madrid (www.oup.es/en).

CONTENTS

ACKNOWLEDGEMENTS   xi

1 What Is the Microbiome and Why Should I Care about It?   1

What Is the Microbiome?   1

Why Should I Care about the Microbiome?   3

What Are Microbes?   5

Who Was the First Person to See Microbes?   9

When Was the Microbiome First Described?   12

What Is Germ Theory and How Does It Fit in with the Microbiome?   14

2 Where Are Microbiomes Found and How Do We Know?   20

What Is the Environmental Microbiome?   20

What Is the Bioaerosol?   21

What Does the Ocean Microbiome Do?   23

What Does the Soil Microbiome Do?   24

vi CONTENTS

Is It Possible to Remove the Microbiome?	25
Can Animals Survive without a Microbiome?	26
How Are Germ-Free Animals Housed?	27
Can a Human live without a Microbiome?	29
How Has Environmental Research Affected Human Microbiome Science?	31
What Is 16S rRNA Sequencing?	33
What Is Metagenomic Sequencing?	35
What Is the Human Microbiome Project?	38

3 The Microbiome and the Skin   41

Are There Microbes in Our Skin as Well as on Our Skin?	43
Is Our Skin an Attractive Living Place for Microbes?	44
How Do We Know Which Microbes Are on Our Skin?	46
Which Microbes Are on Our Skin Right Now?	47
Which Bacteria Are Part of Our Skin Microbiome and Which Are Temporary?	48
Where Do We Get Our Skin Microbiome From?	52
What Happens to Our Skin Microbiome When We Wash?	54
What Is Better, Soap or Hand Sterilizer?	57
Is the Microbiome the Cause of Dermatological Problems?	61

4 How Do Newborn Babies Get Their Microbiome?   64

How Long Does It Take a Baby to Get a Microbiome?	64
How Do We Know What Is Happening?	67
Does the Baby's Microbiome Change over Time?	68
Which Bacteria Are in a Baby's Microbiome?	70
Do Babies Get Their Bacteria from the Mother's Vagina?	71
Where Do Babies Born by Caesarean Get Their Bacteria From?	72

Contents vii

Does Missing Out on Bacteria at Birth Cause Future Health Problems? 73

How Do Anaerobic Bacteria Survive the Transfer? 74

Are Newborn Babies Born Sterile? 75

How Reliable Is Microbiome Research When Studying "Low or No
Biomass" Areas of the Body? 77

How Does the Baby Survive in a Microbial World? 80

Does the Fetal Microbiome Cause Problems for the Newborn? 82

What Are Bifidobacteria? 83

5 The Microbiome and the Gut 86

Should I Get a Gut Test to Check My Microbes? 86

What Does the Intestinal Tract Look Like from the Inside? 88

Which Microbes Are in the Gut? 91

How Reliable Is Microbiome Research? 94

How Do We Get the Microbes in Our Gut? 98

Are There Microbes in Our Tap Water? 101

Do We Get Gut Microbes from our Toilets? 102

Do the Nutrients in Our Diet Affect Our Microbiomes? 103

How Can We Make Sense of the Gut Microbiome If the Microbes in It
Are So Variable? 103

Is There a Core Microbiome? 105

Does Our Gut Microbiome Affect Our Calorie Intake? 107

Do All Animals Have a Microbiome? 108

Can Germ-Free Animals Absorb Their Food Properly? 109

Can We Lose Microbes from Our Gut Microbiome? 111

Does Our Fiber Intake Affect Our Gut Microbes? 112

viii CONTENTS

6 The Microbiome and the Brain — 115

How Long Have We Known about the Link between the Gut and the Brain? — 117

What Is the Gut-Brain Axis? — 118

Do the Gut and the Brain Work Differently in Germ-Free Mice? — 122

How Do We Study the Brain and Behaviors in Mice? — 123

What Do Gut Microbiome-Gut-Brain Studies in Mice Show? — 127

How Could the Gut Microbiome Be Directing the Gut-Brain Axis? — 130

Do Microbial Metabolites Affect the Gut-Brain Axis? — 131

Can Microbes Affect Depression? — 133

Could Microbes Have Evolved to Affect the Gut-Brain Axis? — 135

7 The Microbiome and the Genitals — 138

Why Are the Microbes of the Genital Tract Important? — 138

What Was the Importance of Aseptic Technique When It Came to Childbirth? — 139

What Did Early Research on the Vaginal Microbiome Show? — 142

What Does Vaginal Discharge Consist Of? — 144

Which Microbes Are in the Vaginal Microbiome? — 144

What Do the Microbes in the Vaginal Microbiome Do? — 145

Do Microbes from the Vaginal Microbiome Cause Post-Puerperal Infection? — 147

Are Vaginal Examinations in Pregnancy Still a Recognized Cause of Infections? — 149

Are Lactobacilli Still Regarded as a Key Vaginal Microbe Today? — 150

Do All Women Have Lactobacilli? — 152

Which Lifestyle Factors Can Affect the Composition of the Vaginal Microbiome? — 154

What about the Male Genital Microbiome? — 156

Is the Male Urethra Sterile? — 157

What Is Bacterial Vaginosis? — 158

8 Probiotics and the Microbiome Industry · 161

What Are Probiotics? · 161

What Other Products Does the Microbiome Industry Support? · 163

Where Did the Idea of Manipulating Our Gut Microbes Originate? · 164

What Would Make an Effective Probiotic? · 167

What Are Some Examples of Well-Known Probiotic Microbes? · 168

Are Probiotics Regulated? · 169

What Does the Research on Probiotics Show? · 171

Do Probiotics Work for Antibiotic Associated Diarrhea? · 173

Are Probiotics Safe? · 174

What Do Metagenomic Techniques Have to Say about Probiotics? · 176

What Is a Faecal Microbiota Transplant? · 178

What Is a Clostridium difficile Infection? · 178

What Are DIY Faecal Microbiota Transplants? · 180

Are Any Other Microbiome Therapies in the Pipeline? · 181

What Is the Supplement Paradox? · 182

9 Loss of Microbiome Diversity · 184

What Do We Mean by Diversity? · 184

Is Research on the Microbiome Diverse Enough? · 185

How Is the Microbiome Different between People in Urban Areas
Compared to Rural? · 187

Do Hunter-Gatherers Have a Distinctive Microbiome? · 188

What Is the Cause of These Differences in Microbiome Diversity? · 190

Can Archaeological Samples Tell Us about Microbiome Diversity in the Past? · 192

Can Samples from Other Mammals Show How Our Microbiome Evolved? · 193

Do the Changes in Our Microbiome Diversity Impact Our Health? · 195

x CONTENTS

What Is the Hygiene Hypothesis?	*198*
Can We Rewild Our Microbiomes?	*203*
What Will Future Human Microbiomes Look Like?	*206*

Conclusion 208

Notes	**213**
Index	**234**

ACKNOWLEDGEMENTS

I would first like to thank my editor Sarah Humphreville for giving me the fantastic opportunity to write this book. Her encouragement to "write the book you want to write" really gave me the confidence to grip this project.

I would also like to thank my Dad, Prof John Oxford, both for supporting me during writing, but also for telling me stories of microbes and infectious diseases from a young age. This taught me that if I could enjoy learning about microbes, everyone could.

I would like to thank my book club for their interest and encouragement, especially Aviva Baker, Biomedical Scientist, for her detailed feedback on the final draft. I would also like to thank Dr Peter A Riley, Consultant Microbiologist, St George's Hospital, London, for his expert opinion and kind advice on the microbes of each chapter.

Finally, I would particularly like to thank my husband Anthony for checking every chapter and enjoying endless discussions on the microbiome, so important in helping me develop my ideas.

1

WHAT IS THE MICROBIOME AND WHY SHOULD I CARE ABOUT IT?

What Is the Microbiome?

The microbiome is to do with the friendly bacteria inside our gut. It refers to all the ordinary, healthy microbes that normally live inside us. At the same time as describing the microbes and their generally benign nature, it also describes the home or place where the microbes live—the "biome" part of the word. It implies that the microbes are living together in a defined area: a community of microbes.

The scientific definition of the word "microbiome" is pretty close to our colloquial definition: "the community of microorganisms (fungi, bacteria, viruses) that exists in a particular environment." This word was first used in 1988 in a chapter on fungal parasites by J. M. Whipps et al., who explains that the term microbiome "not only refers to the microorganisms involved but also encompasses their theatre of activity."[1]

There is another definition of the microbiome floating around in the literature: that the microbiome is "the combined genetic material of the microorganisms in a particular environment." This suggests that the term refers only to the microbial DNA and RNA found in a habitat, rather than to the microbes themselves. This mix-up may have occurred because of the dependence of recent microbiome research on genetic methodologies to

2 THE MICROBIOME

detect microbes. We still come across this definition in papers written before 2019, but it has now been officially superseded.[2]

Most people are absolutely aware that we have friendly bacteria inside us. We often come across this information both from adverts on the television or packaging on probiotic foods, explaining that probiotics contain beneficial bacteria. It has to be admitted that cute cartoons with smiley microbes residing inside a neat cartoon image of our intestines does make a change from those spikey, scary-looking germs used to advertise antiseptic kitchen cleaners.

Most people are also aware we have *a lot* of bacteria in our gut, but the idea that there are millions or trillions of microbes inside us is so familiar these days that the shock value has long since been lost. The latest estimate for the number of bacteria inside us is 38 trillion, similar to the number of human cells (30 trillion), meaning the total mass of microbes residing inside us is about 200 grams.[3]

At this point, though, most people's knowledge of the microbiome dives off a cliff. For example, most people don't know that we also have friendly bacteria on our skin. Advertisements for hand soaps that say they remove 99.9 percent of our germs, seem to suggest it is possible, perhaps even usual, for our hands to be microbe free. But the microbes on our hands don't all wash off; many of them live there permanently. And as well as having friendly bacteria in our gut and all over our skin, we also have them on many other mucosal surfaces of our body, our mouths, our noses, our ears, and even our genitals.

A microbiome then can be thought of as a sealed unit with living creatures inside it, a sort of climate-controlled chamber or greenhouse. The Eden Project, a modern botanical garden in Cornwall, United Kingdom, is a very large example of a biome. Consisting of a series of huge climate-controlled domes, like big transparent bubbles cut in half, each dome contains a diverse collection of botanical specimens. There is a Mediterranean biome, a tropical biome, and so on, each with hundreds of plants and even trees from different, warmer parts of the world.

Or a biome could be a sealed and airtight dome millions of miles away, perhaps on another planet. We can imagine the living units that may one day be used for missions on Mars, large inflatable biodomes, sealed off from the planet's atmospheric conditions, designed for astronauts to live and work in comfortably.

Of course, the biomes we are discussing in relation to the microbiome are neither dome-shaped nor conveniently enclosed in plastic. They can be a lot smaller—the microbes in somebody's armpit, for example, or the microbes long dead in a snail's gut in a Victorian museum. Or even smaller than that, the microbes in the midgut of a fly (who knew that flies had midguts?)[4] Conversely, they can be a lot bigger: a ploughed field, a farm, or even a forest. A built construction can have a microbiome too, such as a subway or a hospital.

Almost every single thing we have ever touched has microbes all over it, from the grass in the garden to the sticky hand of our younger brother or sister, from the food that we eat to the bed that we sleep in. There are microbiomes everywhere, in every environment, on every surface, and in every creature.

Many of us may remember with a certain sense of queasiness the day we were first told about germs and that we had millions of bacteria all over our skin. We may remember pausing and trying to imagine tiny see-through germs moving around on our hands. Perhaps we even experienced a sudden squeamish horror at being infested with creatures that we could not see.

Thinking about it now may not be a comfortable sensation either. They really are all over us and on everything we touch. We literally can't get away from them. But if we stay calm and take a close look at the skin on our arms and hands, we will find that it is as clear and as quiet as usual, and with the same smoothness and smell that it always has. We could put the whole idea of microbes and microbiomes out of our minds and pretend that we never knew this information. Or we could find out more.

Why Should I Care about the Microbiome?

We now have an idea of what our microbiome is (all the microbes on and within our bodies) and where we get it from (every surface that we touch), but why should we care about it? That may sound like an oxymoron. We have just said it is everywhere and part of us, so of course we must care

4 THE MICROBIOME

about it. However, we can't see it; for generations, we never knew about it and could quite easily forget all about it.

But if we take a moment to consider, we can see that we can't forget all about it. Our knowledge of germs and bacteria is much more present in our lives than we might think at first glance. We may not necessarily know much about microbiomes, but we all know a lot about germs. From food products to sanitation, from advice on how to live our lives to advertisements on the internet, it turns out that we are considering the microbes in our environment all the time.

"Wash your hands, dear; we don't want germs." "Don't spit; it's dirty." "Irritable bowel syndrome? Maybe probiotics will help." These comments all show a casual but definite awareness of the microbes on our skin, in our saliva, and in our stools. But is the advice right? Should we be washing or using soap this much? Should we be taking probiotics?

"Clean your hands before cooking." Excellent advice again, implying a good knowledge of germs and food hygiene. But does it matter if the food is going to be cooked at 200 degrees centigrade? And how much difference will it make to uncooked food? How many bacteria are on the food we eat each day?

What about toilets? Should the dirtiest item in the house (the toilet) be right next to the item dedicated to getting us as clean as possible (the shower)? For hygiene reasons, perhaps it should be in a separate room. Or maybe it's better for our microbiome if we get a dose of aerosolized stool in the bathroom and accidently swallow it when we brush our teeth.

Lastly, and most confusingly (and most microbiome books appear to be too squeamish to mention this), sex. No matter which school we went to, or in which country, we will have had some equivalent of, or some attempt at, personal and social education by the adults in our lives. This is where as teenagers, we are given very useful growing-up advice and carefully educated about sex, safe-sex, and contraception. But how having sex squared with the handwashing and don't-touch-your-bottom stuff was never fully explained, and no one would ever, ever talk about it.

Hygiene, cleanliness, food preparation, and keeping healthy—these are all areas where we constantly bump into the microbiome and show a genuinely complex knowledge of germs that we perhaps didn't notice we had. But some of the things we have been brought up knowing are true, and some are not. Our knowledge of microbes and our approach to hygiene profoundly affect our microbiomes. It's clear that we do care about the microbiome, even though we are mainly not aware of it day to day, and that's why it's worth finding out more.

What Are Microbes?

Microbes are tiny single-celled microorganisms with a cell wall around them. Little see-through blobs, they live their lives reproducing, consuming organic matter, and eventually dying, just like us.

When microscopes were first invented and microbes were first put under the view finder, nobody knew quite what they were looking at. They could see a mass of different shapes: circles, ovals, and dashes, some of them clear, some of them colored. The scientists of the day began to arrange them into groups, looking at their sizes, their shapes, and their colors—just as we do for larger creatures—to identify, understand, and name them.

At that time, there were only two kingdoms for living things: plants and animals. Microscopic fungi were some of the first microbes to be told apart from the other microbes present, both from their larger size and their distinctive oval shapes (see Figure 1.1). Fungi were designated at the time as plants.

Algae too were identified early. Relatively large single-celled microorganisms, algae contained chloroplasts and could easily be told apart by their colors, bright green or brown. The chloroplasts, which absorb sunlight, showed that algae were also plants (see Figure 1.2).

Protozoa, in contrast, were regarded as animals. Although these were also single-celled microorganisms, many of them were obviously mobile and had distinctive structures designed for propulsion sticking out of their cell walls, allowing them to prey on other microbes (see Figure 1.3).

6 THE MICROBIOME

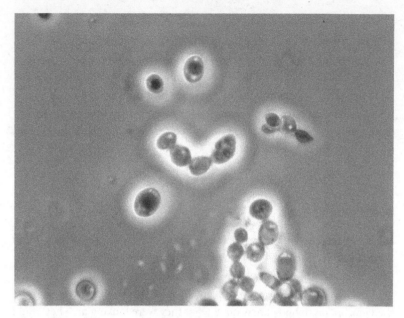

Figure 1.1 Photomicrograph of *Saccharomyces cerevisiae*, microscopic fungi, 5-7 μm in size. These fungi are in the yeast-phase of development, some of which are reproducing by budding.

The word "bacterium" (quite the most numerous and important microbes in our microbiomes) was first coined in 1828. This term was used to refer to a group of much smaller microorganisms: some round, some elongated, some spiral-shaped (see Figure 1.4).

The question was, were bacteria plants or animals? In the first instance, bacteria were considered somewhat similar to algae. Both were unicellular organisms, and both reproduced by transverse division (they divided in half). However, algae had chlorophyll to make energy from the sunshine, but bacteria did not. Also, bacteria were a lot smaller.

Bacteria were also rather similar to fungi or yeasts. Again, both were unicellular, just like algae, but neither had chlorophyll. Yeasts, though, were known to reproduce by budding as well as by division, and bacteria couldn't bud. So, bacteria didn't quite fit with yeasts either.

What Is the Microbiome and Why Should I Care about It? 7

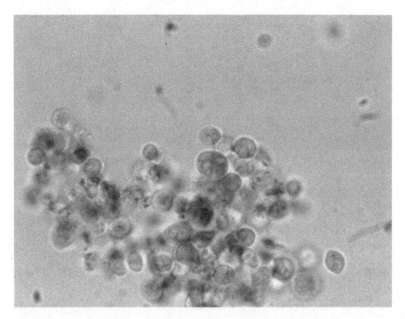

Figure 1.2 Photomicrograph of *Chlorella* sp. algal organisms which vary in size from 2μm-10μm. These spherical-shaped cells contain high amounts of chlorophyll.
Source: Centers for Disease Control and Prevention

From all of the above, we can describe bacteria as microscopic, unicellular "plants" without chlorophyll that reproduce by dividing transversely—a definition that was held to be true until the 1930s.[5]

The final category of microbes that we will discuss here is viruses (including bacteriophages, a category of virus that only infects bacteria) (see Figure 1.5).

Viruses are the smallest of the microbes, famously referred to by Sir Peter Medawar, a fellow of the Royal Society and a 1960 Nobel Prize winner, as "a piece of bad news wrapped in protein." Viruses are so small that it was not possible to visualize them until electron microscopes were invented in 1931, although their presence had been detected long before this using filtration. Viruses are not usually regarded as living organisms because they

8 THE MICROBIOME

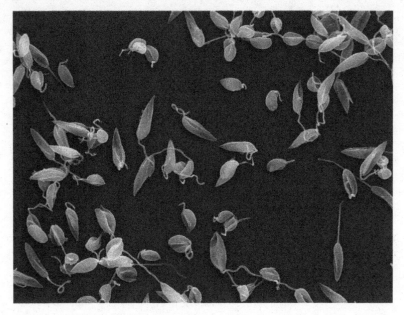

Figure 1.3 Scanning electron micrograph of *Leishmania mexicana*, a unicellular eukaryotic protozoan parasite. These parasites are in the promastigote stage, 15 μm long.
Image credit: University of Oxford, Richard Wheeler.
Source: Wellcome Collection,

cannot independently proliferate and are only able to replicate inside an infected cell.

To get a picture of all these different microbes inside us, we could visualize them as exactly 1 million times bigger than they are in real life. Our single-celled yeast (4 micrometers across) would be an oval shape 4 centimeters across, about the size of a walnut. In contrast, a bacterium (1 micrometer across) would be the size of a hazelnut. Meanwhile, a virus (50 nanometers) would be about the size of a period on this page, tiny compared to the bacteria.

Next to all of these shapes, we have human cells in a variety of sizes: a red blood cell (8 micrometers) 1 million times bigger would be, say, the size of an apple, and a typical skin cell (30 micrometers) would be the size of a throw pillow.

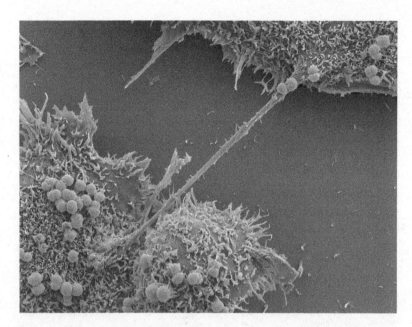

Figure 1.4 Scanning electron micrograph of *Neisseria cinerea* (a diplococci bacteria), 1 μm in size. These bacteria are colonizing the surface of two human epithelial cells, showing the relative sizes of bacteria and cells.
Image credit: Errin Johnson.
Source: Wellcome Collection

We can imagine our hazelnut-sized bacteria floating around our bloodstream, bumping into apple-sized red cells or nuzzling around skin cell sofa cushions, with the occasional period-sized virus and walnut-sized yeast thrown in there, and get an idea of all the sizes of things. Although we can't see these microbes right now, looking down at our skin or our hands, we absolutely know they are there.

Who Was the First Person to See Microbes?

Antonie van Leeuwenhoek (1632–1723), a draper from Delft in the Netherlands, was the first person to describe microbes, which he called "animalcules," after observing them in plaque scraped off his teeth in 1675.

Unfortunately though, for centuries after his death, nobody else could see them because he had kept the technology behind his microscope a closely guarded secret. It was not until the 1820s that microscopes as good as his began to be available once more. These microscopes were then greatly improved by the technical innovations of Giovanni Battista Amici, a microscopist in Italy, and finally, the field of microbiology began to move forward again. As the resolution of microscopes gradually improved from x350 to x600 over the following decades, microbes could start to be distinguished by all.

James Smith of London began producing microscopes in the 1830s. He collaborated with Joseph Jackson Lister, a wine merchant (father of the famous Joseph Lister, the surgeon who first developed the use of carbolic

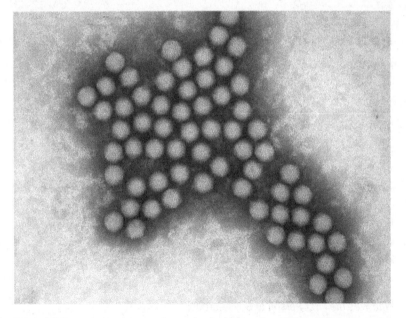

Figure 1.5 Transmission electron micrograph of an Adenovirus, a DNA-containing virus that causes upper-respiratory tract infections. The virus particles are 70–90nm in size.
Image credit: David Gregory & Debbie Marshall.
Source: Wellcome Collection

acid as an antiseptic). Lister knew of Amici's innovation, having traveled extensively in Italy for his business. Together, he and Smith introduced these improvements to London, enabling microscopes to be manufactured to a very high specificity early on and sold to naturalists in England.

For a while following his collaboration with Lister, Smith was recognized as one of the best manufacturers in the country. It's interesting to look at his production rate and consider the slowly growing numbers of scientists now able to access a working microscope. By 1841, he had made a microscope with the serial number 43, six years later he was on serial number 177. By 1863, he had made over 3,000. He advertised them in printed catalogues, offering a range of specs, from £9 and 9 shillings for a simple student microscope to £16 for a superior model ($3,000 in today's money). He even had a range of accessories available, including glass slides and cover slips.

As soon as microscopes began to be widely available, every naturalist and his son must have wanted one. On a quiet, sunny morning, there must have been many gentlemen peering through their microscopes in their front rooms, looking at samples gathered from their gardens and studying the strange little moving dots jiggling about. These early naturalists were looking at samples straight from life. They needed the bright sunshine for their light source, and their microbes were not prepared or stained, but alive, the jiggling due to Brownian motion. We know exactly what these early microscopists could see because they published careful and accurate drawings for other people to learn from, which we still have access to today.

Christian Gottfried Ehrenberg (1795–1876), a German biologist, was one of the first to systematically study microbes. He is still famous for his early classification system. He accurately described many microbes and was the first to identify a 10-micrometer spiral-shaped bacterium, which he named "*Spirochaetes*" in 1838. He also coined the term "bacilli," for rod-shaped bacteria. The spherical, hazelnut-shaped bacteria we mentioned above, later became known as "cocci." Each observation helped the early naturalists to differentiate one species from another and to tell the bacteria from the other microbes; the fungi, the algae, and the protozoa.

12   THE MICROBIOME

The language early naturalists used for microbes was often nonspecific, in keeping with the unknown nature of what they were seeing. Louis Pasteur (1822–1895), born in France and one of the most renowned of microbiologists, was famously muddled in his descriptions of microbes. He sometimes called what he could see "*vegetaux cryptogames microscopiques*" (microscopic cryptogamic vegetation) or "*animalcules*" (little animals), "*champignons*" (mushrooms), "*infusoires*" (infusions from hay allowed to stand with water until bacteria grew), "*torulacees*" (a sort of yeast), "*bacteries*" (bacteria), "*vibrioniens*" (comma-shaped bacteria), "*monad*" (a single cell), "*levure*" (yeast for baking bread), and other terms equally ill-defined. The word "microbe" was not suggested until 1878 by Sedillot (see note 5).

When Was the Microbiome First Described?

The microbiome was first described in 1849 by Joseph Leidy (1823–1891), an American zoologist working in Philadelphia, later to become a leading parasitologist and protozoologist. At the time of writing, Leidy had just finished his medical degree. He had bought himself a Beck's economic microscope (x330) and was reading extensively about "animal and vegetable parasites of living animals." He called these, respectively, "entozoa" and "entophyta" (terms no longer used today), by which he meant parasites and bacteria.

Writing to his friend Spencer F. Baird, secretary of the Smithsonian Institution, he says "From the numerous facts already presented of the presence of cryptogamic vegetation (microbes) in many cutaneous diseases and upon other diseased surfaces I was led to reflect upon the possibility of plants of this description (microbes) existing in healthy animals, as a natural condition. . . . The constant presence of mycodermatoid filaments (types of bacteria) growing upon the human teeth, the teeth of the ox, sheep, pig etc., favoured this idea."[6]

He describes his research on the microbes found on healthy millipedes: "The three genera of entophyte (microbes) of which I have now spoken are all so constantly found in *Julus marginatus* (a sort of millipede) that I look upon it as a natural condition, and should I hereafter meet with an individual without them, I will consider it a rare exception, because in one hundred and sixteen individuals which I have examined during the past thirteen months, in all seasons, and at all ages and sizes of from one up to three inches of the animal, I have invariably found them." He establishes that it is not because the centipede is dead that these microbes are present: he has seen them on living animals and describes three species of microbes, including *Spirillum* and *Vibrio*. He uses Ehrenberg's system of microbe classification, the most up-to-date classification of "infusoria" known at that time.

He concludes, "From these facts we may perceive that we may have entophyte (microbes) in luxurious growth within living animals without affecting their health," and finally, "Thus has been established the law that plants may grow in the interior of the healthy animal as a normal condition and a new field has been presented for the investigation of the Crypto-game-naturalist." It is amazing to think that the microbiome, first described by him all that time ago, is still seen as such a novel and fresh field of scientific endeavor today.

To us, Leidy's reflections on the microbiome seem groundbreaking, but to him the concept of the microbiome was already well established. He modestly remarks, "The recent excellent works by Dujardin, Diesing, and Robin, upon animal and vegetable parasites of living animals render another systematic record of the labours in this field almost superfluous."

Of course, the naturalists of the day did not use the term "microbiome," but rather a variety of other terms that evolved over time, including "cryptogamic vegetation," "vegetable growth," "vegetative bacteria," "commensal bacteria," "avirulent bacteria," "saprophytes," "normal flora," "microflora," and "intestinal flora," among others. It's interesting to notice that all of these terms show a marked and consistent leaning toward a plant-like description consistent with the original classification of bacteria, implying in a delightful way the benign, luxuriant, healthful nature of these flora that many of us still believe to be true of the microbiome today.

14 THE MICROBIOME

What Is Germ Theory and How Does It Fit in with the Microbiome?

Following the discovery of microbes, the idea that microbes lived on healthy creatures appears to have become well known and widely accepted. But germ theory—the idea that specific microbes cause disease—was not yet agreed upon.

Botrytis bassiana, identified in 1837 by Bassi in Italy, was the first-ever microorganism that was proven to cause a specific disease—in other words, a pathogen. This fungus (now known as *Beauveria bassiana*) causes white muscadine, a horrible fungal disease that affects silkworms. When a silkworm is infected, a sort of white powdery substance appears all over them, causing the silkworm to become stiff and moldy before finally killing them.

Although white muscadine was a concrete example of germ theory, this did not yet establish the theory as fact. Germ theory wasn't something that was suddenly established and universally agreed upon, with one scientist's name attached and a neat date. It was an idea that had been thought of long before microbes had even ever been seen, and it took decades of careful experiments before it was fully accepted. This acceptance did not occur until 1876 (and for some people not even then), when Robert Koch (1843–1910), a medical doctor and famous bacteriologist working in Germany, identified the anthrax bacillus, described its full life cycle, and then proved in experimental animals that it, and only it, caused anthrax. Only then was germ theory finally seen as definitely true.

That microbes spread disease is so obvious to us now it hardly seems worth having a theory about. We are bought up knowing from a tiny age about viruses, colds, and bacterial infections. But it wasn't always so obvious. Although more and more microbes began to be identified as pathogens over the course of the 19th century, many prominent scientists repeatedly made the case against germ theory. So, why was germ theory so hard for these scientists to accept?

It's not that they didn't accept the idea that diseases spread between people. This concept—known as contagion theory—has been understood for millennia. During the Athenian plague in 430 BC, for example, one of the first documented plagues in history, it was noted by the Athenian eyewitness Thucydides that caregivers were the most likely to catch the illness, leading to a complete breakdown of society as family members fled and people were left to die alone.[7]

There have, of course, been many, many famous plagues over the past centuries: the Black Death, cholera, smallpox, syphilis, and yellow fever, to name just a few. Each led to attempts by those in charge to reduce spread using methods such as enforced isolation and quarantine. But that did not mean that the people of the time knew exactly how each disease spread or which measures actually worked.

At the same time that Smith of London's microscopes were becoming more widely available, and microbes were beginning to be identified, Sir Edwin Chadwick (1800–1890), the famous English social reformer, published his groundbreaking sanitary report. Although germ theory had yet to be established, as we can see from this document, he was still able to determine how diseases spread.

We can still read all 200 pages of his closely written typescript today, which effortlessly transports us back in time to 1842:

The state of the dwellings of many of the agricultural labourers in Dorset . . . is described in the return of Mr. John Fox, the medical officer of the Cerne union, who, remarking upon some cases of disease among the poor whom he had attended, says: "These cases (of diarrhoea and common fever) occurred in a house (formerly a poor-house) occupied by nearly 50 persons on the ground-floor; the rooms are neither boarded nor paved, and generally damp; some of them are occupied by two families. The up-stairs rooms are small and low, and separated from each other by boards only. Eleven persons slept in one room. The house stands in a valley between two hills, very little above the level of the river, which occasionally overflows its banks, and within a few yards of it. There is generally an accumulation of filth of every description in a gutter running about two feet from its front, and a large cesspool within a few feet behind.

16 THE MICROBIOME

The winter stock of potatoes was kept in some of the day-rooms, and generally put away in a wet state. The premises had not been white-limed during three years; in addition to this state of things, the poor were badly fed, badly clothed, and many of them habitually dirty, and consequently typhus, synochus, or diarrhoea, constantly prevailed.[8]

This is just one eyewitness account among hundreds, gathered from assistant poor law commissioners and medical officers. Chadwick's report showed that damp housing, dirty water, rotting food, and open sewers right by living spaces were associated with high rates of infectious diseases, causing the death of one person out of every thirty-three each year in the poorer districts in England.

Educated Americans looked on closely at England's urban death rates and studied Chadwick's report. When urbanization and industrialization reached the United States, death rates began to match and then surpass England's, reaching one in twenty-seven in 1859. Lemuel Shattuck of Massachusetts—America's answer to Chadwick—report on sanitary conditions (which had been published in 1850), finally attracted the attention it deserved and is now seen as a fundamental document of public health in the United States.[9]

Meanwhile, during the Crimean War of 1854, Florence Nightingale (1820–1910), the English statistician and founder of modern nursing, was working at the military hospital in Scutari, Turkey. She would have been aware of Chadwick's report; indeed, she later worked closely with him. Poor ventilation and miasma (bad air) were thought to be causes of contagion, and this was a theory that Nightingale really bought into. She did not need to know about germs in order to take action. She made it a mission that her sick patients should have fresh air, insisting on open windows and a certain minimal distance between beds to allow air to circulate adequately. She could take strict measures of hygiene, cleanliness, and bed separation, measure the improvement in survival rates in the hospital patients that she worked with, and know with confidence that these measures were helping.[10]

We can feel how close people at this time were to the truth about the causes of infectious disease. They were so close that it almost hurts to hear them debating the matter. We know that microbes can spread by aerosol as tiny floating droplets drifting in the air, easily breathed in; we know they can also spread in heavier droplets that land on surfaces, as well as in water and sewage, and that they are present in rotting food.

But the case for germ theory "was not accepted unopposed, and apart from a vast amount of writing by medical men inadequately equipped for the purpose, many persons of scientific training combated the theory with great ardour."[11]

Some people believed that microbes could just appear out of thin air (spontaneous generation). Others pointed out that only some people got ill from contagious diseases and questioned why that was. Many people did not believe that the various microbes, which were small and hard to differentiate, were separate species. Others thought that microbes could transform into different shapes.

But the major reason for the difficulty in proving that germ theory was correct was, in fact, the presence of the microbiome. If microbes were found in every healthy creature, animal or human, why would it be supposed that they caused disease?

Emile Ducleux, who worked with Pasteur, writes (in French):

The septic vibrio (bacteria) we have said occurs everywhere. Almost always there are billions of them in the intestinal canal of all animals. . . . Why this penetration of the tissues does not occur more often and why the malady induced thereby is not on the list of prevalent diseases is an embarrassing question, and one with which the partisans of the theory of spontaneous generation for diseases should have triumphed. "You see clearly" they might have said "that something more than just the microbe is needed to make us ill, since in this case we so often find the organism and so rarely the disease."[12]

18 THE MICROBIOME

If bacteria caused serious disease, why weren't we all already dead?

What about Leidy's view back in 1849? Where did his newly discovered cryptogamic vegetation in healthy animals leave the germ theory? With astounding elegance, Joseph Leidy sees no contradiction and addresses this point immediately:

> It must not be understood that these facts militate against the hypothesis of the production of contagious diseases through the agency of cryptogamia. It is well established that there are microscopic cryptogamia capable of producing and transmitting disease as in the case of Muscardine, etc., as that there are innocuous and poisonous fungi (see note 6).

In other words, some microorganisms are good and some bad, just as some mushrooms are edible and some poisonous.

Whether other scientists agreed with Leidy or not, the presence of the microbiome meant that every time a microbe was picked out and identified as a pathogen it had to be proved that this microbe really was causing the disease and wasn't just one of the "*entophytes*" or friendly bacteria. Over time, this proof came to be known as "Koch's postulates," as, following Koch's groundbreaking techniques, scientists learned rapidly to identify pathogenic bacteria, isolate them in pure culture, and finally to transfer that specific microbe to other creatures to cause exactly the same disease. Between 1879 and 1900, more than thirty new bacterial pathogens were identified using these methods, utterly transforming our approach to health and disease.[13]

Until now, the focus on pathogens has been right; our understanding of germ theory is an extremely powerful tool to treat and prevent disease. But the microbiome, with its perhaps more subtle effect on our health, also has its place. It's definitely there, and it's starting to become more of an issue. Modern theories of sanitation and hygiene dating back to Chadwick's report have been separating us from our environment and our own microbes for almost 200 years now, through an explosion in the use of soap, antiseptics, and antibiotics. Of course, we want to avoid disease as much as possible, but we must also consider the impact this is having on our microbiomes.

2

WHERE ARE MICROBIOMES FOUND AND HOW DO WE KNOW?

What Is the Environmental Microbiome?

Although this book is mainly about the human microbiome and how it affects us, the environmental microbiome—which includes the microbes all around us, including in houses, in streets, and on the ground, has an effect on our lives too, without perhaps us realizing it. The environmental microbiome is one of the places that we get our microbes from and so is important to us personally, but the activities of these microbiomes are profoundly important not just to us but the whole planet.

Soil science, ecology, environmental microbiology, and oceanography are all scientific specialties in themselves, each with a long and proud history of scientific advances. But each has some important crossover points with the human microbiome. The knowledge of microbes, both in the sea and on land, as well the research technologies developed in these specialties, has had a direct bearing on research on the human microbiome.

Environmental microbiome research is broadly split into three large zones: air, earth, and ocean. There are other environmental microbiome focuses as well, for example the microbiomes of built environments, such as hospitals, subway systems, and homes, and, of course, the microbiomes of other organisms such as plants and animals.

Environmental microbiome research, focusing as it mainly does on those three zones, seems almost mystical or medieval—a bit like Aristotle's four elements, earth, air, water, and fire, so embraced by the doctors of the Middle Ages and even by modern-day pagans. Or perhaps more reminiscent of fairy tale themes, of searching for something. "The Golden Snuffbox" is a good example. In this story, a special and magical item is lost. With the help of the King of the Mice and all his subjects, the King of the Frogs and all his froggy subjects, and the King of the Birds and all the birds, the whole world through is searched (earth, water, and then air), and the object at last is found.[1]

Microbiome research, unfortunately, does not have such a helpful and numerous staff as depicted in "The Golden Snuffbox," but all the same its researchers are making significant inroads into these vast environmental study areas.

What Is the Bioaerosol?

To start with air (after all, it was the eagle, King of the Birds, that found the missing item). This was first studied in 1833 by Charles Darwin (1809–1882), the famous English naturalist, whilst on board the *Beagle*. He documents that on the 16th of January, whilst at sea in the Atlantic, 10 miles off the coast of St. Jago, Jamaica, that "very fine dust was found adhering to the underside of the horizontal wind vane at the mast-head. . . . The wind had been for twenty-four hours previously E.N.E, and hence, from the position of the ship, the dust probably came from the coast of Africa."[2]

Darwin is at pains to point out that he is not the first person to have noticed a dust falling whilst at sea and gives numerous other examples of this phenomena. But it is he who first collected samples of the dust. He corresponded with his friend Ehrenberg, whom we have already met, known for his early classifications of microbes, and delightfully uses the same terms for microbes as Leidy does. "Particles of this size having been brought at least 330 miles from the land is interesting, as bearing on the distribution of the sporules of cryptogamic plants and the ovules of Infusoria." Ehrenberg kindly examined the samples for Darwin under his microscope and confirmed that the microbes present included some infusoria (bacteria), but dried out, and at least two species of algae, one of which he named *Grammatophora oceanica* (still named this today).

22 THE MICROBIOME

It is now well known that sand particles carrying microbes from the Sahara and other areas can be blown long distances in the air. Microbes don't typically float around on their own. They are almost always attached to small particles in the air. If a particle is over 0.7 micrometers in size, then bacteria or fungal spores can attach to it and if under 0.7 micrometers, viruses. In this way, just as Darwin and Ehrenberg surmised, microbes can be blown long distances.[3]

Microbes in the air on dust particles don't seem to have any particular functions, but it is certainly a way for them to move around the globe. Sea spray water particles can also be whipped up by the wind and travel long distances carrying microbes from the sea (see note 3).

Because the microbes of the air are so spread out, so rare in a way, it is much harder to take samples. Air samples suffer from "low biomass" errors, where, basically, there are not enough microbes in the sample to work with. Different devices have been designed to suck microbes in and stick them down in order to get a big enough sample. Other devices have been designed to gather microbes from the air at certain times of day, over successive days, or to measure diurnal changes, proving that there are more microbes present during the day than during the night. Microbes appear to circle around in the lower layers of the atmosphere quite comfortably, but up in the troposphere they thin out, gradually killed off by desiccation and ultraviolet light.

The Victorians, as we know, had a strong interest in the theory of contamination by air and the importance of ventilation. Pasteur, too, was interested in microbes carried in the air and famously took a jar up to the top of the Alps to measure the purity of the air there compared to the city. Although air quality has been somewhat forgotten in recent years in the interests of fire security and also the environment, with tight-fitting doors and windows for insulation, there has been a resurgence of interest in ventilation and air quality recently, and it is clear that there is a real association between microbial counts per volume of air and health.

Air purity measurements of 50–100 microbes per cubic meter are regarded as pure, although the World Health Organization (WHO) recommends that up to 1,000 CFU per cubic meter can be acceptable. Figures like these become important when considering the air quality in a classroom or the packed pediatric waiting room of a hospital, and the balance between ventilation and insulation has started to once again be a point of discussion.[4]

What Does the Ocean Microbiome Do?

In contrast to microbes in the air, those in the sea are much more numerous. Most of us are familiar with plankton, a key set of microbes found in the sea; however, it turns out that the word "plankton" is a catch-all name for sea-based microbes, simply meaning "sea traveler."

Although the early microbiologists classified all living things into one of either two kingdoms, plants or animals, the classification of living things has evolved since then, and the number of kingdoms has increased. Under the domain Prokaryota, bacteria now have a kingdom to themselves: Bacteria. And under the domain Eukaryota, there are now four kingdoms: plants, animals, fungi, and protists.

Plankton includes bacteria, fungi, and viruses, all microbes that we have already met, but it also includes a whole lot of other less-well-classified single-celled creatures that are in the protist group. Some of these are more plant-like, such as algae, some more animal-like such as protozoa, some more fungal-like such as slime-moulds and some have a mixture of characteristics and are known as mixotrophs.

The important thing about plankton is that it is dominated by algae. Algae (now regarded as belonging in the protists kingdom), are microbes especially adapted to the sea, and like plants they contain chloroplasts. This means they are primary producers, getting energy from the sun, just like plants, and starting off the food chain. Algae make more food and more oxygen than all the forests of the world put together. Their effect is massive, and yet, strangely, we mainly don't think about the microbiome of the sea or what it does at all.

Another major constituent of plankton are bacteria, many of which are consuming other cells and degrading organic material into its constituent parts to re-join the circle of life. Bacteria release micronutrients such as iron and magnesium and sequester carbon, allowing it to sink slowly to

24 THE MICROBIOME

the bottom of the ocean. These too are profoundly important actions by the ocean microbiome that we couldn't survive without and yet are mainly unnoticed.

As well as all of these, plankton also includes all the tiny forms of sea creatures such as jellyfish and squid, traveling around in the sea grazing on algae like tiny little herbivores. These are being eaten in their turn by larger creatures such as fish and whales. There are many other strange little protists too, not mentioned here, each one different and many of them displaying predator-like behavior and engulfing other cells when they can get close enough.

Although plankton is thought to make up an amazing 70 percent of the marine biomass within the ocean, these microbes are somewhat spread out—not as much as in the bioaerosol, but still each separated by fifty to sixty body lengths from the other microbes. They are also separated by the different layers of the ocean, responding differently depending on the levels of sunlight, nutrients, and temperatures.

Last of all, let's not forget the viruses and bacteriophages in the ocean, billions in every drop of seawater. In their tiny way, they are often controlling bacteria numbers, which bloom, are then infected by phages, die, and drop to the bottom of the ocean, millions of them. Bacteriophages are thought to kill 20 percent of the bacteria in the ocean every day.

What Does the Soil Microbiome Do?

Soil science, like oceanography, is an entire science specialty in itself. However, the soil microbiome is, in some ways, more similar to the human microbiome than the ocean microbiome or the air and has a closer connection with us too. It too consists of bacteria, fungi, viruses, and protozoa, but not the vast range of other protists and algae seen in the ocean.

Soil and farming techniques have been developed over millennia, and humans have long known the rejuvenating nature of manure, seaweed, and legume crops to improve crop yields and have been using crop rotation since the Middle Ages. Soil science took another stride during the British Agricultural Revolution in the 1750s, and today the findings of soil science and bacteriology have a huge effect on agricultural production. Soil bacteria effect all human and animal food production, as well as the health and biodiversity of every ecological niche in the world, from muddy estuaries to man-made parks. Like the ocean microbiome, it has a perhaps unnoticed effect on our daily lives, in that we don't think about soil microbes except when we come in and wash our hands after gardening or working outdoors.

Bacteria in the soil have just as large an impact on life on the planet as plankton do in the sea, helping with nutrient cycling, breaking down organic matter, sequestering carbon, and recycling key elements such as nitrogen, phosphorus, sulfur, and iron. Soil bacteria also have a key role to play in plant health and live in close association with their roots, fixing nitrogen and enabling the plant to grow better.

Other microbes, too, are associated with plant roots, and together they are known as the rhizosphere. As well as bacteria, mycorrhizal fungi also have a very close relationship with plant roots, acting as an extended root system for the plant, increasing growth by up to 50 percent and reducing the chance of soil pathogens taking hold. Bacteria in the soil are not spread out as they are in the air or the ocean, but live shoulder to shoulder and in close communication, heavily reliant on each other.

Of course, it's not all about microbes in soil science, just as it is not all about microbes in human health. Soil characteristics and plant growth are affected by many different aspects such as soil type, soil microstructure, organic materials, temperature, moisture, pH, and contaminants such as salt, azo dyes, and nitrogen runoff, among many others.

Soil qualities explicitly affect human and animal health, which in turn profoundly affects the soil. This is now being acknowledged with the "One Health" movement, which started in 2004, bringing together veterinary scientists, wildlife conservationists, and medical scientists. The microbiome continues to be a key crossover point between all these different specialties.[5]

Is It Possible to Remove the Microbiome?

Since the invention of microscopes, we have known the microbiome is there, on every creature and on every surface. But over the 19th century, as the specialty of bacteriology began to get established, a discussion began to

26 THE MICROBIOME

occur in scientific circles about whether it would be possible for an animal to live without its microbes.

Pasteur played an important part in this discussion. Well aware of the "trillions of bacteria everywhere," he thought it would not be technically possible to live without a microbiome. Or if it did become possible one day, that an animal would not be able to survive. "For several years during discussions with young scientists in my laboratory I have spoken of the interest in feeding from birth a young animal with pure nutritive products which have been artificially and totally deprived of the common micro-organisms. Without affirming anything, I do not conceal the fact that I would undertake such a study with the preconceived idea that under these conditions' life would become impossible."[6]

Many scientists agreed with Pasteur then, and some even today, that even if a sterile living chamber could be designed, it would be impossible for an animal to survive without microbes. But others simply wanted to test the idea. The very first germ-free animal chambers were developed in 1896 by George Nuttall (1862–1937), an American bacteriologist, using steel canisters.

Can Animals Survive without a Microbiome?

The development of germ-free animal chambers allowed scientists to attempt to raise an animal, born by caesarean section, in a sterile environment. By achieving this landmark step, Nuttall was then able to prove that animals really could be reared in a germ-free environment, proving Pasteur wrong. It turned out that it was possible for an animal to survive without a microbiome.

To begin with, germ-free creatures did not thrive. At first, it was hard to work out if the differences between germ-free creatures and conventional ones were due to the lack of microbes or simply the result of inadequate diets, housing, or management. But once the difficulties in formulating sterile but nutritious food were sorted out, it was found that animals could live without a microbiome.

In fact, germ-free animals tended to be slightly larger, glossier, and livelier than conventional ones. They had well-groomed fur and bright eyes. They even lived longer, with male germ-free mice on average living 723 days compared to 480 days for conventional ones. It was clear that these animals looked alright, but were they really okay?[7]

From the start it was obvious that having no microbiome affected certain organs. Organs that did not come into contact with the microbiome were pretty much the same, such as the brain and the heart, but others were smaller or thinner than usual, such as the skin, the small intestine, and the lung alveoli.

The large intestine, the organ with arguably the most contact with the microbiome, was markedly affected. The cecum, the sac that forms the first part of the large colon, was especially enlarged in mice, up to eight times as big as usual, sometimes making it difficult for the animals to walk or even leading to premature death. Without bacteria to break down plant material, it was thought that the remaining cellulose in the colon absorbed water, swelling and causing this enlargement. Symptoms were much relieved by the addition of sterile fiber to the diet, showing that fiber is essential even in the absence of a microbiome.[8]

How Are Germ-Free Animals Housed?

Today, germ-free animals are still being used in science, and some scientists see them as key to microbiome research. But they are expensive and only found in highly specialized laboratories. Even if they are obtained for an experiment, it doesn't take more than one mistake to turn them from germ-free animals to a perfectly ordinary animal with plenty of microbes on it, no longer useful for research. Instead of the stainless steel that Nuttall would have used, transparent flexible PVC is now used to make isolation chambers.

To keep the animals germ-free, these centers need a very, very meticulous lab technician and a rather particular range of equipment. There needs to be a fan going the whole time so that there is positive air pressure in their containers, so that if there is a leak, air is blown out rather than microbes sucked in. The fan needs an air inlet, an air outlet, and, of course, a filter.

There has to be arm-length gloves attached to the cages to manipulate items within the cages such as water bottles and waste or even to handle the animals themselves. There needs to be autoclave-resistant supplies such as bedding and food and a sterilizable supply canister to put the supplies into, ready to transfer them into the chambers. There has to be a dock on the chamber for the supply cylinder to attach to, usually using a PVC sleeve, and a way of sterilizing the docking joint. Different methods of sterilizing include an autoclave (which uses heat), irradiation, or the use of sterilizing chemicals.[9]

To confirm that the mice are still germ-free, there has to be regular testing for microbes on the bedding, the food, and the stools, usually every four weeks. The mice are held to be sterile "as far as we know" or "to the best of our testing ability."

If you have visualized the mice in a series of transparent plastic bubbles, each resting on a counter in a windowless, white-painted room—perhaps even with a gowned and masked technician arm deep in stiff black gloves changing their bedding—now consider a human in this situation.

Everything is present, just as for the mice: a sterile PVC living space, loud fans going on day and night, and an autoclaved steel supply canister docking intermittently with containers of sterilized food. The large, elbow-length black gloves are there too, sticking out of the surface at intervals, but this time the technicians are nurses, the setting is a hospital in Texas, and the PVC bubble is big enough for a baby to lie in.

This was the situation David Vetter was in as a newborn baby. Born on September 21, 1971, he had severe combined immune deficiency (SCID), a genetic condition that meant that his immune system was profoundly abnormal, meaning that he couldn't survive more than a few days without protection. As he entered the sealed chamber in which he was to live until the end of his life, he became "the boy in the bubble"— later made famous by Paul Simon's song.

Can a Human live without a Microbiome?

At the hospital in Houston where David Vetter was born, as well as a team of immunologists, there was a gnotobiologist researcher named Raphael Wilson, who was trained in germ-free research at the University of Notre Dame. Wilson was a Catholic brother, sometimes listed in research papers as Br. Wilson, and later accused of sexually abusing two boys.[10] Wilson somehow persuaded the family to deposit David, seconds after his caesarean birth, into a prepared sterile container, triumphantly announcing to the hospital staff, "I've got my baby." David remained here until less than two weeks before his chaotic death on February 22, 1984, at the age of twelve.

In the view of Raymond J. Lawrence, who was involved as an ethicist in the case, "This project was demonic at its core and should never had been carried out in the first place and must never be repeated." Strong words, but hard to disagree with once you have read a full account of David's life.[11]

In 1971 (and possibly still; it is not recorded that he has died), Wilson apparently saw David as "observational research." He published at least two papers on David in 1973 and 1974, with or without his permission (presumably without) and writes in one of his publications, "The continued maintenance of this patient in a gnotobiotic state has provided opportunities for serial studies in an uncomplicated disease state."[12] By the time David was four, Wilson, although nominally David's "godfather," had abandoned the "project" and left.

So how did being germ-free affect David, a human boy? David appears to have been an articulate and intelligent person who developed normally, according to the account written by one of his main caregivers, Mary A. Murphy. However, being stuck permanently in a bubble did alter David's perception of the world. For example, among numerous strange ideas, he could not be persuaded that the buildings he viewed from his window were three-dimensional. Nor did he believe that anything existed below the surface of the Earth, even when shown a plant and its roots. And he could never understand the difficulty of crossing oceans, believing that the surface of the sea was as firm as the ground was.

He never sat but only squatted or knelt; his diet was baby food. He never ate any fresh fruit or vegetables and didn't even have a pencil for many years because of the difficulty of sterilizing it. His mental health was severely affected by being enclosed, and he often had nightmares about "the king of germs" attacking him. He could be found frequently sucking his thumb and rocking, reciting "1, 2, 3, 4, I can't take this anymore," and sincerely believed he "should have been allowed to die age 3 when he would not have known about death or what was killing him."

According to Lawrence, many adults who saw him were "speechless and horrified to witness a human being trapped indefinitely in a sterile chamber." His parents would today be seen as key decision-makers, and it could be argued that they did not make the key decisions at the right times for David's best interests, whomever they were persuaded by (Wilson certainly had a hand in this). According to Lawrence, they remain committed, as did many of his doctors, "to an idealised portrait of David as a heroic little boy who contributed much to medical science." It would certainly be preferable for this narrative to be accurate and that there was some point to his suffering rather than no point at all, but it is difficult to be persuaded by this description (see Figure 2.1).

As David is the only germ-free human who has ever lived, or rather the closest we will ever get (and it is to be hoped that his experience will never be repeated), and as a person who could speak for himself, we find he was okay without a microbiome. He not only survived but was, in fact, healthy. Despite the best efforts of his team, microbes did enter his enclosure. By the age of four, there were thirty-five bacteria and seven yeasts in his enclosure, but no viruses or protozoa.

It was the enclosure, not the lack of microbes, that appeared to have caused David's perceptual problems, his mental health decline, and his severe and never-ending distress. Many children die in tragic circumstances, and at David's own hospital at that time, there were terminally ill children; he was even friends with some of them. But there is something about David's situation that is especially dreadful: about being trapped, about being used as a scientific subject without his permission, and about the adults

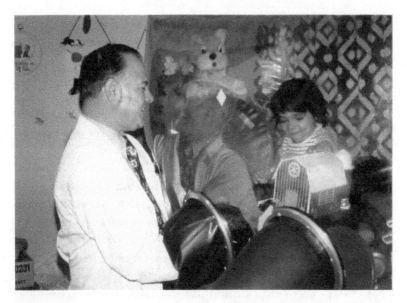

Figure 2.1 David Vetter with John Montgomery, his pediatric immunologist.
Author: Michelle Goebel

nearby who allowed it. We can now only acknowledge his life with respect and hope that he rests in peace.

Germ-free animals are not in the real world. We have evolved to live cheek by jowl with microbes, to have microbes all around us constantly, and to cope with this contact safely. Germ-free animals, in their microbe-free world, cannot properly demonstrate the processes that we depend on day-to-day that allow us to safely come into contact with and even consume microbes. But studies on germ-free animals can be informative, even though they cannot tell us the whole story, and we will come back to germ-free animals and the effect being microbe-free has on their health later in this book.

How Has Environmental Research Affected Human Microbiome Science?

We have stepped away a little from environmental microbiomes to discuss these completely germ-free environments, a concept in a way completely

32 THE MICROBIOME

opposite to that of a microbiome. But we now return to ocean environmental research, as scientific innovations in this specialty have had a huge impact on human microbiome science.

These innovations really started in 1992, when two different teams of ocean environmental scientists, Fuhrman and DeLong, both used a technique called 16S rRNA sequencing and identified a highly unusual type of microbe called *Methanomicrobiales* in a sample of seawater taken from the Sargasso Sea.[13,14]

Although known about since 1956, *Methanomicrobiales* was initially thought simply to be a rather unusual sort of bacteria, one that could live without sunlight but that processed other chemicals to get energy, such as sulphur. To start with, these microbes were only found living in environments with extreme temperatures such as in hot pools or by hydrothermal ocean vents, and for this reason are often known as "extremophiles." It was only in 1977 that, using very early genetic techniques to sequence the DNA of these microbes, a scientist named Carl R. Woese realized how different they were from normal bacteria. They were so different that he realized that they were not bacteria at all, but examples of an entirely new domain of life forms. He and his colleagues coined a new term for them: "archaebacteria."[15]

It may feel strange that we have gotten this far in the book before revealing a whole new sort of microbe, but as you can see, this new domain is relatively new in science too, and it took time for the news to percolate through the scientific world. When it did, the term "Archaea" was used instead, on the grounds that these microbes were so completely different from anything else seen before that they shouldn't be named after bacteria.[16]

So now all the organisms of the world are divided into three domains: Bacteria, Eukaryotes (plants, animals, fungi, and protists), and Archaea.

When in 1992 these two scientific teams separately announced that they had identified *Methanomicrobiales*, a species of archaea in ordinary well-oxygenated, well-lit water floating about in the Sargasso Sea, it overturned all previous knowledge about these microbes. Not only had scientists found that there were archaea present throughout the ocean, but they had also found that they were numerous, accounting for over 2 percent of the microbes in the ocean. If archaea could be found in ordinary water, where else could they be found? And with 16S rRNA gene analysis, what else could be found?

What Is 16S rRNA Sequencing?

16S rRNA sequencing, the technique that Fuhrman's and DeLong's teams used, is a genetic technique that allows microbes to be identified in samples just from their genes, without the necessity of having to see them under a microscope or to try to culture them. It is an absolutely key technique and still used very frequently in microbiome research.

The term "16S rRNA" refers to the name of a gene. Because this gene is so important, it is found in all bacteria. The "rRNA" stands for ribosomal RNA. Ribosomes are key to a bacterium's survival because they help bacteria synthesize proteins.

Because the gene is so important, many parts of it are exactly the same in every bacterium, and these parts are called "highly conserved." But other parts of it are variable and completely different in each species. It is these sections can be used to tell one bacterium from another. As an added advantage, this gene is not in human cells, and so there is no confusion there (although we do have our own version: 18S rRNA).

Fuhrman's and DeLong's teams looked at all the different versions of the 16S rRNA gene that they could find in their seawater samples. The DNA sequence of every single version was then written down and compared to a library of sequences. This allowed them to work out which bacteria were present. As *Methanomicrobiales* was so difficult to identify by sight or culture, it might never have been found in these samples without this technique.

Following these two environmental studies, 16S rRNA sequencing techniques totally captured scientists' imaginations and took the environmental world by storm. It wasn't long before researchers working on human samples also began to borrow this new technique, finding hundreds of novel bacteria and even archaea in the human digestive track too.

But although a powerful and exciting advance, this technique is not perfect. Errors can creep in at every stage, from obtaining and preserving a

34 THE MICROBIOME

sample on a research vessel out at sea, to the computer that matches the sequences back in the lab. Even simply releasing the genetic material from tough bacterial cell walls can be fraught with problems: if the sample is broken up too much, it fragments into tiny unusable pieces; if not enough, then not all the genetic material is extracted.

There are many discussions about which computer programs to use when analyzing the sequences, which gene library to reference, and how to interpret the findings. For example, if a DNA match is 97 percent identical to a library sequence, this is conventionally presumed to be good enough to securely identify a bacterial species. But some scientists suggest the match need only be 96 percent identical. Conversely, some microbes (such as *Escherichia coli* and *Shigella dysenteriae*) have identical 16S rRNA genes. Even though they are thought by most to be completely different species, they can't be told apart by this technique. As well, this technique excludes viruses and fungi, which do not have a 16S rRNA gene.

Another disadvantage is that although 16S rRNA sequencing will prove that a gene of a bacterial species is in a sample, it cannot tell if that microbe was dead or alive when it was collected or reliably how many were present. This may not be so important when used in an environmental sample, but it is very important in a human sample, especially when taken from a part of the body normally regarded as sterile or where a microbial presence is regarded as rare. The numbers and proportion of each microbe present can tell us a great deal about the significance of each. To have an extensive list is fantastic, but to have no idea of each microbe's frequency is a limiting factor.

Meanwhile, environmental researchers had rushed on. Within ten years, a scientist named Venter published another groundbreaking technique based on a sample of seawater from the Sargasso Sea: shotgun metagenomic sequencing.[17] Using an early sequencing machine called the ABI 3730XL DNA sequencer, in 2004, Venter's team identified 148 previously unknown bacterial phylotypes, proving unheard-of levels of oceanic microbial diversity.

Before we think about shotgun metagenomic sequencing, you might be wondering, as an aside, why oceanic science again and why the Sargasso

Sea again? How could it be featuring so prominently in environmental microbiome research for a second time? This is a good question, and the reason appears to be because of the unique ecological nature of the Sargasso Sea (bounded on all sides by a clockwise flow of major ocean currents). It attracts scientific researchers and is supported by the Bermuda Institute of Ocean Science (BIOS), which has driven new scientific techniques at an amazing rate.

We can imagine Venter aboard the RV *Weatherbird II*, skimming over the ocean in the Sargasso Sea one quiet evening in February 2003. As the sun sets, he leans over the side and reaching as far as he can, scoops up a sample of seawater in a sample bottle. Screwing on the lid and shaking off the sea spray, he labels it carefully "Hydrostation S."

Of course, it didn't happen exactly like this. The sample was a "surface water sample" and the quantity "170 litres," and as Venter explains, "sampling protocols were fine-tuned from one expedition to the next." The samples were then combined, and shotgun metagenomic sequencing was carried out.

What Is Metagenomic Sequencing?

Metagenomic sequencing is a technique that analyzes not just one gene, but every single little piece of DNA within a sample, identifying all of the microbes present: fungi, viruses, and bacteria (but not RNA viruses).

If that sounds like a lot of work for one sample, that's because it is. And it's only possible because of modern sequencing machines. As pioneers in this technique, Venter's lab had developed their own sequencing machine, enabling them to break new ground in metagenomic sequencing in 2004. The first commercially available machine, Pyrosequencing 454, made in Connecticut, became available in 2005, and later machines include Illumina (2006) and Ion Torrent (2010). Each machine had different efficiencies, costs, and quirks, and as new machines have continued to be developed, they have become cheaper, faster, and more accurate, revolutionizing microbiome research.

36 THE MICROBIOME

Metagenomic sequencing has different names, and at first glance, it can seem as if each term is referring to a different technique, when, in fact, they all describing the same thing. Terms include "next-generation sequencing," "second-generation sequencing," "shotgun sequencing," "whole metagenomic shotgun sequencing," "deep sequencing," "high-throughput DNA sequencing," and, lastly, a personal favorite, "massively parallel DNA sequencing."

Just like 16S rRNA sequencing, the DNA has to be extracted from the cells and purified. It then has to be broken down and separated from its matching pair, as the machines can only process small sections of single-stranded DNA, down to 100 base pairs.

The different names used for this kind of sequencing are quite illustrative: "massively parallel" describes the hundreds of microwells where the DNA fragments are being processed—all in rows and in parallel, all being sequenced. And "shotgun sequencing" conveys the idea of randomness, the chopped-up bits of DNA being sequenced randomly but at the same time.

Of course, this technique gives a ton of sequencing data for each tiny sample, so the final stage of metagenomic analysis is making sense of all this data, all these small pieces of DNA sequence now written down. Analyzing a big set of biological data like this is sometimes called bioinformatics; it takes time and specialized computer programming to sort through it all.

Each short little bit of DNA has to be stitched together in the right order using overlapping pieces of sequence using programming, and this gives us a whole read of a particular microbe's DNA. A complete read may enable scientists to identify the microbe by name or even to identify that this is an entirely new microbe, never described before.

Metagenomic sequencing analysis doesn't stop here. With modern molecular biology techniques, each full DNA sequence can then be analyzed to give a list of all the potential genes that might be transcribed (metatranscriptomics), all of the proteins that a particular microbe might make (metaproteomics), and even which metabolites it could potentially synthesize (metabolomics).

More recently, a technique called "nanopore sequencing," a tabletop device, has also started to be utilized as well. It can process much longer pieces of DNA much more quickly (although admittedly with a very high error rate) but can be used to help scaffold and stitch together the DNA and get overall more accurate readings. It is also starting to be used experimentally alongside standard protocols in clinical testing for infections.

Although these techniques sound powerful (and they are), they still may not always be the best way to study an organism. If, for the sake of comparison, we took the DNA of a human (which we actually already did in fact; the Human Genome Project was completed in 2003) we still wouldn't really know a lot about humans—not even what a human looked like. One of the quirks of the Human Genome Project was that even when this amazing goal had been achieved and the entire human genome transcribed, we still didn't know very much, not even which parts were genes and which parts were dead space or redundant DNA.

So as an approach, the "omics" have their strengths (they shed light on the whole microbial community) but also their limitations. Just like 16S rRNA analysis, we don't know if any of the organisms detected are alive or dead, and we don't know how many of each microbe is present. And when a microbe new to science is discovered using this technique, we can't study it in real life, because all we have is a readout of its chopped-up DNA.

But it didn't matter. Following Venter's thrilling discoveries, every environmental scientist was fascinated. Among the soil scientists, many "found it virtually impossible to resist the attraction of genomics techniques then being developed and increasingly used in biological research."[18] It wasn't long before these techniques started to be applied to human samples too. Unheard-of levels of diversity and microbial numbers began to be identified in the human digestive tract.

The volumes of data crunching and analysis needed in these new techniques were astounding. It was soon realized that these programs needed to be properly developed and databases shared. It was more or less exactly at this time and for these reasons that scientists, with the help of the Obama administration, established the Human Microbiome Project.

38 THE MICROBIOME

What Is the Human Microbiome Project?

"The potential for discovery is staggering . . . the opportunity afforded by metagenomics to study microbial communities in their natural state represents an endless frontier."[19]

In 2007, following the developments in metagenomic science and their increasing application both in the environmental sciences and in medicine, the National Research Council (NRC) commissioned a publication on metagenomics. The publication was a well-written, exciting, and enthusiastic description of "The New Science of Metagenomics" and must have been highly persuasive. The American government agreed to invest $215 million to research the human microbiome using metagenomics. The NRC was commissioned to set up the Human Microbiome Project (HMP), which it did as a collaborative research project, shared among different institutions in America.

The Human Microbiome Project, in some ways the starting place of modern microbiome research, was accomplished in two phases: HMP1 from fiscal years 2008 to 2012 and the integrated HMP (iHMP) from 2013 to 2016. When HMP1 was launched, it was much lauded for its emphasis on having a large sample group and rigorous longitudinal follow-up. When we realize that HMP1 studied just 242 Americans, sampled only twice, we might think that this applause was slightly exaggerated. However, given the complexities of metagenomic research, for the time this was an extremely large sample size. Previous studies had been restricted to two to three subjects, gradually stretching to around fourteen in one large project on obesity.

The HMP1 subjects were both male and female, between the ages of eighteen and forty, of whom 20 percent identified themselves as a racial minority, but the key aspect of this group is that they were carefully selected to be *healthy* individuals. The whole point of the HMP1 was to characterize a normal, healthy microbiome.

The HMP1 was highly successful in many of its goals, which were not only to describe the healthy microbiome of the gut, the skin, the mouth, the airway, and the genitals, but to also establish standardized methods and protocols and to set up an open-access library to store the findings, the Data Analysis and Coordination Centre (DACC).[20]

The iHMP, in contrast, following five years later, focused on three *disease* areas: diabetes, inflammatory bowel disease, and the vaginal microbiome—in order to try to link the microbiome with a disease process and further try to understand what the microbiome actually did, rather than just what it looked like.[21]

Lita Proctor, former HMP coordinator (and, interestingly, before that specializing in oceanography) agreed that studies focusing on the function of the microbiome were important: "Interventions that could help treat . . . diseases will be discovered only if we move beyond species catalogues and begin to understand the complex and mutable ecological and evolutionary relationships that microbes have with each other and with their hosts."[22]

As well as funding the HMP, the American government then invested another $728 million into hundreds of smaller microbiome projects. Finally, it commissioned an investigation into how the money had been spent, which analyzed every research project that had been sponsored, illustrating the breadth and depth of this microbiome research as well as its wild expansion.[23]

The HMP has been a huge project, and although it has now ended as a funding project, microbiome research has continued to expand exponentially and worldwide, with over 20,000 papers published in 2020 alone. Many countries, including Canada, Japan, the United Kingdom, and those in Europe, have been inspired to launch their own microbiome projects. As scientific techniques have progressed it has enabled these projects to become larger and more ambitious, often including a longitudinal aspect planned to last for many years to try to tease out the links between the microbiome and our health. The goal of these studies is to find out not just what the microbiome looks like but also what it actually does, including its effects on our nutrition, our immune system, and whether it is implicated in disease.

Of course, in a book like this (or indeed in any book), we cannot hope to cover every avenue of research that the microbiome has reached into, but we can consider the main import of microbiome discoveries and focus

40 THE MICROBIOME

in more detail on such areas as the gut, the skin, and how we get our microbiomes in the first place. Ultimately, our focus is on what is called "translational microbiome science"—applying what we have learned about the microbiome in a concrete and practical way to human health, but we will come across many fascinating aspects about the microbiome on the way.

3

THE MICROBIOME AND THE SKIN

The skin microbiome is the first human microbiome that we will take a really close look at in this book and in some ways, it feels like a very accessible part of the body to study. We can easily glance at our skin right now as we read. The thousands of microbes on the surface of our skin, are, of course, perfectly invisible to us. But although we can't see the microbes, we are seeing their environment, the "biome" of the skin. We can feel its warmth and flexibility, detect its smell of salt or sweat, and know if our skin is moist or dry. These aspects—temperature, dryness, saltiness, and oils—make up the skin's biome and have a bearing on which microbes can survive.

These parameters also help to create a variety of habitats for the skin microbes to live in, broadly divided into three zones: dry, oily, and moist. This is a division that may be familiar to many of us, having read it scores of times in magazines trying to persuade us to buy cosmetics. But it's really true: hands and arms are examples of the fairly dry parts, faces and heads examples of the more oily or greasy parts (being well supplied with sebaceous glands), and the axilla (armpits), groin areas, and skin folds, profusely supplied with sweat glands, are the most sweaty or moist habitats.

As well as this, each part of our skin has different amounts of contact with the environment. Some areas of our skin are almost always kept covered with clothes; in contrast, other areas are almost always out in the sunshine and the wind. Consequently, our skin obtains, retains, or alternatively sheds microbes at different rates according to each site.

Because of its accessibility, the structure of the skin has been extensively studied. It has a well-described structure consisting of three layers that we can easily visualize. The epidermis, the outermost layer of our skin, is the layer that we touch. Under the epidermis is the dermis, which contains the hair follicles, nerves, and sebaceous glands. Below the dermis is the adipose tissue (the layer of fat), which we can sometimes feel under our skin as a padded and more mobile layer. Because these layers line up so neatly, the skin is usually illustrated in a cross-sectional view, like layers of a rainbow cake. Each layer is usually depicted in a different color: we can visualize a narrow buff-colored strip for the epidermis, a wider pink layer underneath it for the dermis, and under that another wide layer, this time colored yellow for the fat.

For us, the top layer of the skin, the epidermis, is our microbiome habitat of interest and therefore the focus of our attention. This structure also has its separate layers. The bottom part of the epidermis (resting on the dermis) is the stratum basale, a sort of membrane. This has a nice, simple single layer of oblong keratinocytes neatly aligned all over it. Keratinocytes are the key cells forming our epidermis and are produced continually at this membrane by cell division. Some of these cells stay at the stratum basale to continue dividing, but others are pushed upward toward the skin's surface.

The epidermis is basically formed of layers and layers of keratinocytes. Among the keratinocytes, there are also melanocytes (pigment cells) scattered about and Langerhans cells (a special sort of immune cell). As the keratinocytes move up toward the surface over a leisurely four to six weeks, they undergo a process called "keratinization," whereby they get progressively more and more keratin inside them, making them strong, flexible, and waterproof. As they travel (or are pushed upward by fresh cells coming in), they change shape from that initial oblong shape, and become gradually more spiky looking. The spiky shape enables them to make tough bonds with each other, and this helps to create a strong skin barrier. The cells then excrete lipids to fill the gaps in between, and this keeps the skin barrier watertight.

As the spiky keratinocytes approach the surface, they get gradually flatter, finally losing their nucleuses altogether and becoming known as

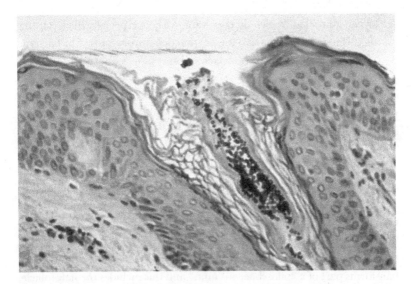

Figure 3.1 Photomicrograph of a skin section showing the layers of the epidermis. The middle portion of the image shows an infected hair follicle in which the hair root has been infiltrated with characteristic, spherical, yeast-form cells; a fungal pathogen.

"corneocytes." These now dead cells form the stratum corneum, the outermost layer of our epidermis, formed of about fifteen layers of corneocytes. These cells are renewed continuously, and the entire layer is completely replaced about every two weeks. That dead surface of the stratum corneum is the surface that we can actually touch and indeed touch with.

By the time the corneocytes reach the very top surface, they are only 1 micrometer thick and are ready to be shed as squames. When magnified, these squames look like old, dried leaves, or scales, or discs of poplar bark, and they slough off our skin surfaces throughout the day, taking with them any attached microbes (see Figure 3.1).

Are There Microbes in Our Skin as Well as on Our Skin?

If we imagine a nice, sliced potato dish made with layers of potato, laid flat on one another, where the oval potato slices represent layers of corneocytes, it's as if some erroneous cook has willfully scattered peppercorns throughout the layers, more than you could ever want, with an especially thick crusting on the surface of the potatoes—the peppercorns representing our bacteria.

Microbes are all over the surface of our epidermis just like the peppercorn crust. They land daily on our dry, ready-to-shed corneocytes and squames and try to make a home and a living for themselves. Just as in our potato dish, they are found on the surface and throughout the fifteen, flat dead layers of the stratum corneum. However, they don't get much further. They don't really get past this to the spiky layers of the keratinocytes below, and they certainly don't get through that bottom layer, the stratum basale, unless there has been a breach of the skin.

The dermis, the layer underneath the membrane, is essentially sterile, except for a few discrete areas associated with hair follicles. The tips of our hairs, of course, stick out well above the surface of our skin, but the root of the hair plunges right down through stratum basale into the dermis. Each hair forms part of a "pilosebaceous unit," and this includes the hair follicle, an associated sebaceous gland to keep the hair shaft oiled, and a pilo muscle to make our hairs stand upright when we are cold. Microbes can, and do, travel from the surface of the skin, down the hair follicle, and into the sebaceous gland, where they live in a nice anaerobic microenvironmental niche. But not always; the pilosebaceous unit can be sterile too.

This association of microbes and hair follicles has not only been proved by microscopy but by electron microscopy too. In 1969, a series of beautiful electron microscope images of skin sections were published that demonstrated microorganisms in the most superficial layers of the stratum corneum but mostly clustered around the upper parts of the hair follicles.[1]

Is Our Skin an Attractive Living Place for Microbes?

If we think about our skin in an ecological way, as islands or territory in a world teaming with microbes, we can see that it is territory that needs to be settled. In many ways, though, our skin is not an attractive living space for microbes. The defining characteristics of our skin that we mentioned above means that this habitat is a sort of dry, salty, cold, and arid kind of plain, reminiscent of the dried-out salt flats high up in the Andes of South

America. Any microbes that have succeeded in settling on our skin have had to adapt to these (for microbes) extreme conditions.

Our skin is cooler than the rest of us, only 32 degrees centigrade (compared to our core temperature of 36.7 C). It is dry because of the dry, dead corneocytes, and because of this is very unlike the moist habitats that bacteria usually like to thrive in. It is bombarded by ultraviolet rays, especially our face and hands, acidic from the lipids excreted from the cells and salty from our sweat. Keratinocytes are hard for bacteria to digest (most microbes can't cope with them), and the lipids that the keratinocytes produce, as well as being acidic, are also antimicrobial. Most of all, the keratinocytes and corneocytes keep on moving upward, and the squames keep on shedding, so that although a bacteria may feel like it's found a foothold, it might suddenly find itself flying off into the air like a paraglider unintentionally jumping off a cliff.

Because of this continual, natural shedding of skin cells, each of us is, in a way, a walking cloud of microbes. We shed squames and their attached microbes everywhere we go. A study of skin flora performed in the 1960s found that healthy individuals exercising naked (in the interests of science) in a sterile room for thirty minutes, each dispersed 2 to 6 million viable organisms.[2] And a more recent study on the inhalable bioaerosols of an underground subway network noted that the most common bacteria present in the air breathed in by people on the platforms were those associated with human skin—reaching a peak during rush hour.[3]

Although we started off this book talking about "friendly bacteria," from this description it doesn't look as if the skin sees bacteria as particularly friendly at all. The acidity, the salt, the lipids, and the shedding are all arranged to discourage and kick off bacteria. These strategies are constantly decreasing the number of bacteria on the skin even without washing. It has been proved that even if we spit on our hands (adding several hundred million bacteria to the skin surface), an hour later most of these organisms will have disappeared, "even though the hands have not been washed in the interim."[4]

Because of these innate defenses and this rather hostile environment, the density of viable bacteria on the skin is rather low, at 1,000 to 10,000

46 THE MICROBIOME

per square centimeter, not in the millions. But bacteria are tough. They have a hugely faster generation rate than humans and have adapted and learned to love these dry, cold, salty, airy plains and the sparse diet of sebum and keratin.

How Do We Know Which Microbes Are on Our Skin?

William H. Welch (1850–1934) was an American surgeon and bacteriologist writing in Baltimore in 1895, and as the discoverer of *Staphylococcus epidermidis*, he is particularly important with regard to the skin microbiome. As a surgeon, he had a special interest in skin bacteria and a deep concern about surgical wound contamination.

By this time, as well as using microscopy to identify different microbes, bacteriologists like Welch had an increasing number of other methods to identify bacterial species. Microbiome samples could easily be collected from the skin using swabs or scraping the skin with a sterile blade. Once obtained, these samples could then be cultured and stained to identify which bacteria were present.

Culturing a pure sample of bacteria is still a key technique, developed by Koch in 1875. The further development of staining then allowed microbes to be seen more clearly under the microscope. To grow or culture bacteria, agar gel (a sort of clear jelly) was poured into specialized flat-bottomed glass saucers with lids (petri dishes). When set, the jelly formed a smooth, flat surface for the bacteria to grow on.

If a skin swab of bacteria was then lightly brushed over the gel, it sowed a scattering or streak of bacteria on the gel's surface. Where just one viable bacterium was seeded, pure cultures of bacteria would grow, and these were known as a "colony." These colonies, each 2 to 3 millimeters across, look like little colored buttons in white, pink, or yellow, just the right size for a small doll to use. The distinctive appearance of each colony allowed scientists to differentiate bacteria still further. With pure cultures, the individual characteristics of each species could then be described and identified.

At this time, the synthetic dye industry was also taking off, with many new and amazing aniline dyes. As soon as it became obvious that some dyes selectively stained certain cell structures or species, these were rapidly assimilated by bacteriologists to further aid identification. One of the most important of these was, and still is, the Gram-stain. Made of an aniline dye called "gentian-violet," it was found to stain some bacteria a deep purple. These species became known as "Gram-positive bacteria." Others did not retain the purple dye when washed out by a decolorizing agent and were stained pink by the counterstain. These became known as "Gram-negative organisms."

From the first, it was noticed that the Gram reaction correlated with various important bacterial characteristics. Only later was it realized that it was the bacterial cell walls that were being stained; the Gram-positive species indicated thick cell walls, and the Gram-negative species thin ones.

Which Microbes Are on Our Skin Right Now?

Because our skin is our interface with the environment, it is obvious that there could be an extremely wide variety of microbial species found here. Welch was well aware of this. "As the skin is exposed to contamination from the air and all sorts of sources it is evident that there is scarcely any limit to the number of species of bacteria which may possibly be found on the skin. Most investigators of this subject have not had the patience or have not thought it worthwhile to attempt to identify or to describe all of the different kinds of bacteria developing from the surface of the skin."[5] However, as if in exact contradiction to Welch, metagenomic scientists really have tried to detect every single bacterium on our skin.

Our skin microbiome is dominated by bacteria, which account for over 80 percent of the microbes present. These are almost always Gram-positive aerobes. The thick cell walls of these bacteria allow them to cope well with the dryness and oxygen-rich conditions of the skin.[6] The most numerous are *Cutibacterium* (formerly known as *Propionibacterium*), *Corynebacterium*, and *Staphylococcus*, but there is a long tail of other less-numerous bacteria picked up of all sorts, including Gram-negative anaerobes such as *Enhydrobacter aerosaccus* and *Veillonella parvula*.[7] If we look more closely at the different skin habitats of the body, we find that each habitat supports a different set of bacteria. The moist, sweaty areas of our body tend to have more *Corynebacterium* and *Staphylococcus*, the greasy areas *Cutibacterium* and *Staphylococcus*, and the dry areas such as our hands an extremely variable set of bacteria of all sorts.

Archaea account for approximately 2 percent overall, including *Thaumarchaeota* and *Euryarchaeota*.[8] Fungal species for about 5 percent, including *Malassezia, Aspergillus, Rhodotorula*, and *Candida*. Viruses are also abundant, especially bacteriophages that attack *Staphylococcus* and *Cutibacterium*. The usual wart-causing pathogens such as Human papillomavirus, Molluscum contagiosum, and Merkel Cell polyomavirus are also present (see note 7). Any one person can have over 100 different species.

However, as we can see, simply listing the variety of microbes found on the skin does not convey that much. The number of species found on each person is very large and the combinations vary considerably from one person to another. We may be feeling a bit baffled at this point. Some of these bacteria may be important to our health, and some may be completely irrelevant. How can we get a handle on what the presence of all these bacteria means?

Which Bacteria Are Part of Our Skin Microbiome and Which Are Temporary?

A meaningful microbiome is not just the microbes found on any one day but the microbes living in a *stable* relationship with the host. It is the long-staying microbes that we are interested in. These are the ones that we may have a "relationship" with. The difficulty is telling which microbes are long-stay residents and which are temporary.

We can infer that a microbe is probably a resident if we repeatedly recover it in large numbers. But how do we discriminate between minor residents and transients? And are all residents good and all transients bad or is the picture more complex than this?

If we return to our arid, salty plain in need of settlement, let's assume that it does now have a settled and stable community, like a village perhaps, or a small town. In a similar way to any community, this small town has a diverse variety of inhabitants. Some are residents and live here long term (bringing up families, holding down jobs), but others are transients and stay only for a short time before moving on.

Many of our long-term residents may be thought of as benign members of the community. In contrast, many transients could be seen as a bad influence, drifters and opportunists. But neither of these assumptions is necessarily correct. Some residents, it is true, appear to help out in the town with gardening, law and order, and obtaining nutrients. But others, just like in an Agatha Christie murder mystery novel, having lived in the town for many years, perhaps even been regarded as pillars of the community, if given the opportunity can cause serious problems. In contrast, many transient members are perfectly benign individuals and cause no problems, or even are just what the community needs and may end up settling and becoming a resident.

"Transients" and "residents," "pathogens," and "benign commensals" are all terms we use for microbes in their habitats. "Mutualists" is another, a term that refers to two organisms that live together, both benefiting from the arrangement. Just as in the above description, not all transient microbes on the skin are "bad" pathogens, and not all resident microbes are benign.

An example of a known pathogen is *Streptococcus pyogenes*. This microbe can cause very severe skin infections, and other serious infections too. It is almost always a transient pathogen. Another typical pathogen is *Pseudomonas aeruginosa* (formerly known as *Bacillus pyocyaneus*), a bacterium famously known for producing a blue pigment, hence its original name. Both of these bacteria are on the PATRIC (Pathosystem Resource Integration Centre) list of pathogens and listed on the Bacterial and Viral Bioinformatics Resource Centre (BV-BRC). These are good examples of the sort of bacteria that, if we ever came into contact with -perhaps through patient contact—we would wish to wash off right away.[9]

In contrast, many *Staphylococci* species are known benign skin commensals or residents of the skin and don't seem to do us any harm, for example, *Staphylococcus aureus*. One less-benign version of *S. aureus* that you may have heard of though is MRSA (methicillin-resistant *Staphylococcus aureus*). This is an antibiotic-resistant variety of *S. aureus*. This bacterium is assumed by most people to be harmful and most of us would not want to carry MRSA in

50 THE MICROBIOME

our noses or our groins. However, you may be surprised to realize that 20 to 40 percent of us do carry it and seem to be perfectly alright. MRSA, therefore, can be seen as an example of a transient pathogenic bacterium that can sometimes become a resident and cause no harm—or it can become a resident and do a lot of harm.[10]

In contrast, another species of staphylococcus is called *Staphylococcus epidermidis* and has completely different qualities. This is a well-known commensal bacterium, intensively studied. Welch, our surgeon, proudly identified and named this species in 1891. "Although in general, the bacterial flora of the skin is inconstant and indefinite in its special characters, there is one bacterial species, to which I gave the name of *Staphylococcus epidermidis*, which is found in such regularity in cultures from the skin that it may properly be regarded as a regular inhabitant of the normal skin" (see note 5).

S. epidermidis is indisputably one of our long-stay residents, and some would argue one of our "friendly" bacteria. In common with all the *Staphylococci* species, it is well adapted to the harsh environment of our skin. It is able to adhere well, thrive in cool temperatures, tolerate salt, and digest keratin. It is also known to produce antimicrobials that actively discourage other bacteria such as MRSA from colonizing. So its presence on our skin may actually protect us from pathogens. This is an attribute known as "colonization resistance"—an important attribute of the microbiome that we will come back to throughout this book.[11] Unfortunately, the chemical nature of this antimicrobial factor or factors that *Staphylococcus epidermidis* harnesses, while recognized as a known function of some bacteria today, is still unidentified.[12]

The effect of colonization resistance on our health with respect to our skin, although well recognized and certainly real, could be supposed to be relatively small. It is our immune system that does the heavy lifting in protecting us from infections, as we can see clearly in patients with a compromised immune system. For example, in end-stage HIV infection, we don't see the skin bacteria fighting off invading pathogens; we see the exact opposite. Minor fungal and viral pathogens, such as the causes of seborrheic dermatitis and molluscum contagiosum, —infections that wouldn't normally get much of a toehold—manifest as significant skin infections.

Many claims have been made about the "function" of *S. epidermidis* and the mutual benefits it may provide us, such as promoting skin healing and tolerance to infections. But can a bacterium like *S. epidermidis* really be this friendly and this useful? Or is it like our Agatha Christie suspect, living quietly and without reproach in the village for many years and turning murderous when given the slightest opportunity? Because although *S. epidermidis* usually lives quietly all over every one of us, if it does breach the skin barrier, just like any other bacteria, it will cause an infection.

None of this duality about the nature of *S. epidermidis* is news—or rather, it shouldn't be. In science, sometimes we rediscover things that were known 100 years ago. Welch, the discoverer, was well aware. He writes in 1895, "*S. epidermidis* is usually innocuous. . . . However it can cause stitch abscess and it is prone to travel down along the sides of a drainage tube, and under these circumstances may cause the wound to suppurate." And in 2023, Severn, a microbiome scientist, concurs with apparent surprise but an almost identical description: "*S. epidermidis* remains one of the most frequent causes of implant-associated infections in the United States, and these antibiotic-refractory, biofilm-associated infections are costly for patients and the healthcare system."

So, *S. epidermidis* appears to be both a mutualistic commensal and a pathogen depending on its circumstances—on the one hand, a seemingly helpful and ever-present member of the skin community, but on the other, a destructive criminal if given the chance.

It's fun to anthropomorphize microbes and think of them settling a territory and getting on in a small town together, and trying to work out if *S. epidermidis* is the good guy or the bad guy. But if we take the analogy too far, of course, it can lead to misinterpretations. A transient microbe such as MRSA is neither a motorcycle-riding drifter come to make trouble for the town nor a newcomer who wishes to set up a helpful community project for the homeless. Microbes really are just tiny blobs that will multiply if given appropriate nutrients and temperatures.

And although we are describing our microbial skin inhabitants as living in "communities," which for humans is seen as a good thing (implying cooperation and helping out for the common good), when it comes to microbes, we shouldn't necessarily see them as kind and beneficent, living together in

52 THE MICROBIOME

harmony. We instinctively want to when we hear the word "community," and maybe, possibly, some microbes like *S. epidermidis* do provide us or each other with some benefits. But microbes are not friendly. They are not even usually friendly to each other. Many of them produce antimicrobials to discourage other bacteria from moving in and taking over the territory. They are just there, ready to proliferate if they can, or not, if times are hard.

We live in a world thronged with microbes, and our immune system has evolved to cope with that situation. Our skin literally can't stop microbes settling on it. But as we have seen, it has developed numerous mechanisms to keep microbes at bay, including our constantly replenished fifteen-cell-thick layer of dead skin cells all over us as a sort of barrier or interface, almost like a magical repellent or defensive force field. We are obliged to tolerate the microbes on our skin, and it seems that for humans to be mainly settled by a bacterium such as *S. epidermidis* may be the least bad option.

Where Do We Get Our Skin Microbiome From?

We get our skin microbiome both from our environment and from each other, principally through the medium of contact or touch. Our hands, feet, elbows, and some other parts of the body have a lot of contact with the environment. In contrast, other parts, such as our armpits, have almost none. But out of these, it is our hands that probably have the most contact of all. It is our hands, as key transmitters of our skin microbiome, that we will focus on particularly.

Hands provide a secure conduit of movement for the microbiome, a highway if you like. They move microbes from our face to our feet, from our genitals to the environment (and back again), and from person to person, all through constant touching, handshakes, and hugs.

Whenever we touch something (or someone), we are picking up microbes and also depositing them.[13] Analysis of our homes and even our pets demonstrates this constant sharing of microbes. It is known that, over time, living in the same house, people's skin microbiomes become gradually more similar, even more so if they are partners and sharing a bed. The fixtures and fittings of our homes reflect this too; the microbes found on our light switches, doorknobs, and kitchen surfaces all showing a resemblance to the microbes found on our hands.[14]

If we analyze how often we touch things during the day, we find that we are touching some kind of external environmental surface such as keyboards and tables about 90 percent of the time. A study that was done in China, conducted specifically to measure these kind of touch episodes simply videoed an office of thirty-nine postgraduate students (with their permission). It then analyzed every single touch episode that occurred over five full days. It was found that as well as touching external objects, students also touched themselves extremely frequently, on average ninety-eight times an hour. Not anything inappropriate or intimate: over 50 percent of these touches were to their hair, face, neck, or shoulders (designated as HFNS for the purpose of the study). This must be something that we are all doing all of the time but that we don't notice or simply don't see. If we ever thought how many times a person might have touched themselves before we shook hands with them, we would be horrified. Actually, though, we shake hands frequently with perfect strangers and are fine.[15]

Our right hand is much more likely to touch the right side of our face and our left hand to touch the left, but our dominant and nondominant hands act in different ways. Over 63 percent of touches of external and environmental surfaces are made by the dominant hand, and in contrast, the nondominant hand makes over 66 percent of the self-touches to the HFNS -including to the mucous membranes for tasks such as eye rubbing and nose picking.

The different activities of the two hands somewhat account for the differences in right- and left-hand microbiomes. Our hands typically harbor over 150 unique species, nearly two-thirds from just five genera: *Proprionibacterium*, *Streptococci*, *Staphylococci*, *Corynebacterium*, and *Lactobacillus*.

As well as different touching habits, the microbes of our hands are affected by all sorts of other things, such as handwashing, cosmetic use, food preparation, and the local environment. There are differences between men and women, with *Proprionibacterium* and *Corynebacterium* being more abundant on men and *Lactobacillaceae* more abundant on women. There is also typically a greater diversity of species on women's hands.[16]

Because hand microbiomes really are so distinct between individuals, it was initially proposed that a person's microbiome could be used for forensic identification. The idea being that metagenomic sequencing would allow a phone to be matched to its owner or could identify a criminal's movements from traces left on a light post or a café table. However, unlike fingerprints or human DNA, which are stable for a person's entire life, the skin microbiome varies so much within the same person, sometimes shifting within hours, that it was found in trials that people could only be reliably matched to a neighborhood surface swab 50 percent of the time (and then only within a short time frame), indicating that this technique would have a limited application at best.[17]

What Happens to Our Skin Microbiome When We Wash?

The effect of washing and the utility of handwashing is especially interesting for doctors as well as for many other healthcare workers, as it has a direct effect on their lives, not just daily but hourly, and as well, a direct impact on the lives of their patients. In fact, for a family doctor seeing six patients an hour and washing their hands between every patient, this impact may occur every ten minutes.

One of the most thorough pieces of research ever carried out on handwashing was published in 1938 by Philip B. Price, a surgeon working in Baltimore. Price researched hand-washing for nine years. As a surgeon working at a time before antibiotics, when cleanliness was everything, he *really* wanted to know which bacteria were on his hands and exactly how many. His work was influential, and his recommendation that surgeons scrub their hands with brushes under running water for seven minutes still guides the development of surgical handwashing protocols and WHO guidance today.[18]

Price came up with a novel way of measuring the number of bacteria on his hands. Instead of using skin swabs, agar gels, or glove juice, Price found that by washing his hands in a sterile bowl in a known quantity of sterile water, he could measure the number of viable bacteria in a sample of that water. "By plating and culturing measured specimens of the water, counting the colonies, and multiplying by total volume, the exact number of bacteria removed can be calculated." This important measurement is known as the "colony forming unit" (CFU). This technique, measures the number of each bacteria instead of just the number of different species. It tells us critical information about the numbers of each species that metagenomic sequencing is often unable to match.

Price's techniques are exact; he delineates the soap used, the types of water (hard, soft, or distilled), the brushes to scrub with (moderately stiff and sterilized), and time allowed to soap and scrub to the elbow (forty-five seconds) (see note 4).

We can imagine a series of enamel basins (fourteen, in fact) all lined up on a workbench, each containing an identical volume of sterile water. Price is there wearing old-fashioned surgical greens, scrubbing his hands and arms at each bowl in turn. There is a gowned and masked assistant nearby to help with passing towels and equipment.

By culturing a small sample from each basin of this now-dirty water, he worked out the bacterial totals. He calculated that in the first basin he would typically wash off approximately 500,000 viable bacteria. The number of bacteria per basin gradually diminished, so that by the fourteenth he would typically wash off only 100,000. When plotted on a graph, his measurements gave a smooth and predictable curve, reliably re-created every time he repeated the experiment. After the experiment was over, he found that it took seven days for the bacteria on his hands to return to normal numbers.

Using this technique, he proved that each of us has approximately 7 million bacterial residents and 1 million transients on our hands. Scrubbing for two minutes removed practically all of the transients. By eight minutes, it was possible to reduce the total bacterial load to 3 million, but, of course, he

56 THE MICROBIOME

was never able to remove them all. Price's work proves—not unexpectedly—that it is impossible to sterilize our hands. Some people say that his work illustrates the apparent fruitlessness of handwashing—that there is always a reservoir of unreachable bacteria within the stratum corneum.[19] However, it is clear that Price understood the normal microbiome of the hands well. His goal was to improve the safety of surgery by fully understanding the effect of handwashing, not a futile or foolish wish to remove all hand bacteria.

Price relates fascinating anecdotes about his practice of medicine in the 1930s. He describes how on one occasion he was "in active charge of a ward full of patients with virulent infections following gunshot and shell wounds." In spite of his usual frequent and thorough hand scrubbing, he unfortunately picked up a series of pathogens, including *Bacillus pyocyaneus*, as it was called then, the bacteria with the blue pigment. This bacterium then became part of his resident hand bacteria—sometimes at very high levels. For a time, it accounted for over 50 percent of his total bacterial load and "did not disappear from the hands for many weeks after the writer ceased work on the septic ward." As a result of this experience, he advises that pathogenic contaminations should be removed from hands promptly and completely. "Otherwise, there is a danger, not only of immediate spread of infection, but that these hands may become chronic carriers of pathogenic bacteria."

"Transient bacteria appear to lie free on the skin or are loosely attached by grease and other fats along with dirt . . . (and) . . . are removed with relative ease by washing with soap and water." Price was the first person to describe the concept of transient bacteria and the first to prove the efficacy of handwashing in getting rid of them.

We can't see on a daily basis when we wash our hands what Price managed to see with his equipment, his serial basins, and his constant plating up and culturing. Our hands often look clean both before and after washing them. Instead, we have to constantly work our imaginations. We have to imagine what microbes we might have picked up and added to our usual hand microbiome. We have to imagine them being transferred to other surfaces if we are not careful. Then, more satisfactorily, we have to imagine them being loosened off with soap and water and washed down the drain.

What Is Better, Soap or Hand Sterilizer?

A quick and unstudied answer might be that recent evidence suggests alcohol gels are better. But alcohol gels are not always the best choice, and for many of us, they are not our go-to hand cleaner.

Any occupation or profession that needs frequent handwashing—not just in healthcare but also in food preparation, working with young children, or simply working in the home—relies on handwashing to prevent infections, and for this, it has proven effectiveness. But there are problems. Handwashing is a constant drain on time and resources, and people don't always feel like washing their hands. Sometimes they don't have the right equipment, sometimes they are too busy, and like anything, sometimes handwashing doesn't work.

Handwashing (over forty times a day for some workers) can feel distressingly uncomfortable or even painful. This is because soap causes a number of harmful changes to the skin. It increases the pH of the skin, making it less acidic and less antimicrobial. It reduces the lipids produced by the skin, leading to increased transepidermal water loss, and it can lead to the loss of antimicrobial effects of the lipids. It causes skin reddening, increases desquamation, and disrupts the skin barrier, leading to greater microbial shedding.

In fact, it affects every aspect of the skin's functioning, causing changes that are present for days—as Price proved. Keratinocyte lipids do not return to their usual levels for at least three hours after washing. Skin damage and dermatitis can become chronic, making the skin less resistant to pathogenic microbes and permanently altering the skin microbiome—for the worse.[20]

Healthcare workers are advised to "decontaminate" their hands before touching a patient, after touching a patient, before a procedure, after a procedure, and after touching a patient's surroundings. These are known as the five "points of contact," and this important mantra is repeated to healthcare workers at frequent educational meetings. But to advise healthcare workers that they could potentially be washing their hands five times per patient, as well as being impractical, may end up being counterproductive. It is well known that healthcare worker's hands have more pathogens on them, including MRSA, *Candida albicans*, and *Enterococcus* species, because of frequent washing and skin damage.[21]

It may be that we have reached the point of diminishing returns with continued campaigns to increase the frequency of handwashing as currently practiced. So, how do we square this circle?

The first point to mention is with regard to the concept of cleanliness. The point of handwashing is not just to reduce the number of microbes on our skin; we can see there is no point in that. The great majority of the microbes on our skin are part of our microbiomes. They are securely interleaved between our corneocytes and cannot be washed off. A better aim for handwashing is to remove the transient pathogens, just as Price advised, not just a bulk reduction in microbes. But the overall goal is not just to reduce the numbers of pathogens on our hands but to reduce the incidence of actual disease, such as gastrointestinal infections, diarrhea, and respiratory illnesses.

The WHO recognize this key outcome measure of disease reduction in their handwashing guidelines, but they come up against a hard place when trying to assess different handwashing products. Most assessments of the efficacy of a new product are made by simply measuring the change in the number of microbes left on the hands five minutes after use. Where a product says, "Kills 99.9 percent of most common germs," it's true; they really do kill 99.9 percent of microbes. But the reason they pick that number for their advertising is because according to the Food and Drug Administration, a product is not allowed to be listed as an antimicrobial product *unless* it reduces the bulk number of microbes by 99.9 percent. But don't get too excited by this efficiency. First of all, as we have already established, we don't care that much about the bulk reduction of microbes. And second, if we start out with 8 million microbes on our hands as Price suggests, that still leaves 8,000 knocking around, plenty to be getting on with.

It is difficult and expensive to test real-world reductions of gastrointestinal infections or respiratory illnesses as a result of a better handwashing product. At least 6,000 participants would be needed just to measure a 2 percent change in incidence, a reduction from say 7 percent to 5 percent. However, scientists have tried. Using the best testing methods that we can, it has become clear that alcohol gel (of at least 60 to 80 percent by weight) is the most effective hand-cleaning agent. It causes less skin irritation, it's easier to use, and it clears away at least as many, if not more, microbes than soap and water.

It's as well to be upfront about what alcohol gel is not so good at. It is not as good at clearing away protozoa and viruses. And it is no good at all at killing bacterial spores (important when talking about spore-forming pathogens such as *Clostridium difficile*). Just to be clear, soap and water doesn't kill bacterial spores either, but it does wash them away. Nor can alcohol gel clean away actual dirt or blood or other contaminants, for which soap and water is still essential. But overall, alcohol gel has not only been proven to reduce the spread of infections; it has also improved efficiency and efficacy in healthcare settings, being quicker and less resource-heavy than soap and water. It has also improved handwashing compliance.

Somewhat naively, WHO or various public bodies (or, anyway, someone) thought that alcohol gels were so good that they would arrange for them to be available to the general public. This would "promote change" and improve health in one simple step. For a while (and some readers may remember this), alcohol gel hand sanitizers could be seen everywhere—in public rest rooms, in schools, and in railway stations. Everyone had free access to them—although, strangely, they often seemed to run out very quickly or even disappear overnight.

And then a number of reports of alcohol gel poisoning started to emerge. National poisons agencies noted a doubling of unintentional poisonings in children and a doubling in intentional ingestion by experimenting teenagers. Adult alcoholics were also found to be deliberately drinking the hand gels.[22] Even in the carefully monitored environment of a hospital ward, intentional oral ingestion by in-patients occurred. In one case, a 53-year-old alcoholic on ICU, unbeknown to the team, ingested "several

60 THE MICROBIOME

containers of alcoholic foam hand sanitiser," lost consciousness, and had to be intubated for twelve hours. It did not take too long for these sanitizing products to be rapidly removed from most public places.[23]

Alcohol hand gels have their place, and we use them in many settings, but for many of us, soap and water is still the best handwashing agent. Any soap is good, whether solid or liquid. Solid soap should be allowed to dry out between uses. If it is liquid soap, the soap canisters must not be refilled. (A study of bulk-soap-refillable dispensers noted the horrible fact that over 25 percent of dispensers in public restrooms were contaminated with *Klebsiella pneumoniae*, *Enterobacter*, and *Pseudomonas* spp.) So, single-use liquid soap canisters only please.[24] Lukewarm or cool water is best and patting dry with paper towels (rather than rubbing): both of these measures are important and cause the least skin damage. Drying carefully is essential as wet skin propagates the spread of microbes. Paper towels are preferred to air driers, which are thought to aerosolize microbes. Finally, a skin emollient applied after washing significantly mitigates skin damage and reduces microbe shedding.

In a home context, antibacterial soap products are usually best avoided. This is because we know bacteria tend to get resistant to antibacterial chemicals. Although washing regularly with antiseptic soap does initially lead to less bacteria, bacteria that are resistant to the soap soon find a foothold, and the numbers of bacteria on the skin then go up again. Typically, the usual bacteria do eventually return (but ones resistant to the soap). This pattern is repeated with any antibacterial products, including antibacterial solutions, antiseptics, and antibiotics. When washing most parts of the body, rinsing with plain water is usually best, and antiseptics, soap, and, especially, shower gel are better avoided.[25] If we don't wash at all, it doesn't necessarily make a difference to the overall number of bacteria present. When the skin on the shoulder blade is kept unwashed for seven days, the skin pH goes up a little, and the salt detected on the skin from sweat increases very slightly, but the numbers of bacteria, usually 100 per square centimeter, stay more or less the same during that period (see note 11).

There is no doubt that hand-washing interrupts the transfer of microbes on that busy highway of microbial transfer supplied by our hands.

It may even reduce that microbial connection that our hands usually give us between the different microbiomes of our bodies, between us and our environments, and between each other. However, as well as the positive effects of removing pathogens and significantly reducing the transmission of infectious diseases, we have seen that there are negative effects of hand washing in that it damages our skin barriers. But it may also be altering our microbiomes. Not just the ones on our hands, but also microbiomes in many locations of our bodies. We will come back to this important concern and also consider other lifestyle measures that may be having an impact on our microbiomes throughout this book, but particularly in the last chapter, where we discuss microbiome diversity and its effect on our health.

Is the Microbiome the Cause of Dermatological Problems?

There are many skin conditions that microbiome scientists have focused on in the hope of finding a relevant application to healthcare, including acne, chronic wound infections, aging, psoriasis, rosacea, and many others. As yet though, no obvious link has been found, and microbiome research in these areas has not yet translated into clinical advice. However, if we were to focus on just one condition, perhaps a key concern or interest for many of us is the effect that the skin microbiome has on atopic dermatitis (or eczema as it is usually known).

There has been an interest in the normal flora of the skin and its relationship to eczema from the earliest days of bacteriology. This has been discussed at dermatology meetings at least since 1893, with much talk of "care of the soil" or "terrain." It was felt, right from the start, that if the skin was well cared for (just like any garden), the right flora would flourish. Indeed, it was felt that the real concern might be almost the opposite: that of how to "restrain the fertility of the extensive flora dermatologica," as it had already been noticed that overgrowth of certain bacteria was associated with eczema or dermatitis.[26]

Paul Gerson Unna (1850–1929), a dermatologist from Germany and an early researcher of the skin microbiome (or what he called the "cryptogamic flora of the skin"), described in detail the "existence of a large number of

62 THE MICROBIOME

species of microbes" on the skin. He was famous for his book *Histopathology of Skin Diseases* and was the first to differentiate seborrheic dermatitis (a sort of flakiness typically found on the eyebrows and around the nasal flares) from other sorts of eczema. He also elucidated the cause of seborrheic dermatitis: *Malassezia*, a fungal species, commonly found on the skin and easily treated nowadays with antifungals. Hope was therefore high at this time that a microbial cause for eczema might also be identified.

But dermatologists were critical of Unna's research, pointing out that he was not differentiating between "the bacterial forms actually living on the skin, and germs accidently present as they might be on any surface exposed to the air." This is the same difficulty that Koch, Welch, Price, and all the early bacteriologists faced (and that today's microbiome researchers still have): working out which of the bacteria present on the skin are relevant to human health and which are not, differentiating pathogens from the microbiome.

"Are these organisms saprophytic inhabitants of the skin, or are they introduced from without? Are they capable of producing eczema . . . or is some preliminary disturbance of nutrition necessary for them to exert a pathogenic effect? Or may these, therefore, be only accidental contaminants which might be removed without the morbid process coming to an end?" J. F. Payne writes, convener of a skin flora dermatology meeting in 1897.[27] There was "no difficulty whatever in finding bacteria" on the skin during bouts of eczema, he continues. "There are only too many of them, but the problem is to pick out those that are truly pathogenic."

But careful observation of the natural history of eczema makes it obvious that this condition, instead of demonstrating the "saprophytic growth, local virulence and finally active contagiosity" consistent with an infective cause, demonstrates the exact opposite. Symptoms are typically symmetrical, rashes spring up in distant parts of the body (the elbow creases, knee creases, wrists, or the neck), and it is never contagious. It is often associated with asthma and hay fever, and it is typical to find a family history of the condition. The cause at the time was felt to be a family predisposition or a "special vulnerability" of the skin, theories that are still agreed with by doctors today.

But hope springs eternal, and microbiome researchers 130 years later—aware that bacteria like *S. aureus* and *S. epidermidis* (as we know, both normal constituents of the skin microbiome) bloom during a flare of atopic dermatitis—are still studying these microbes closely. They still conclude that "the functional role of staphylococci in driving the atopic dermatitis disease state is poorly understood," and undeterred, are still calling for more research, suggesting that "longitudinal sampling at more frequent intervals before a flare" should be carried out "to identify whether increased staphylococci levels precede clinical symptoms . . . rather than bloom in consequence of it" (see note 7).

But if eczema were caused by microbes, then doctors would surely have cured it by now using antimicrobial medication. A well respected review combining the results of forty-one studies to study the use of antibacterial agents for eczema found them completely ineffective.[28] It seems likely that the skin microbiome, although affected by eczema, is unlikely to be the cause. Knowledge of the microbiome in this instance is unlikely to translate into any transformative treatment for this condition.

4

HOW DO NEWBORN BABIES GET THEIR MICROBIOME?

Every time a baby is born, it's a remarkable moment. With every birth, a completely sterile baby comes out for the first time ever, into a world brimming with microbes and yet it survives.

It's a bit like taking our germ-free animal out of its sterile, ventilated chamber and just letting it loose in a grassy field, out into the real world. It's as big a deal each time as if we took David Vetter, but a David with an intact immune system, carefully out of his PVC bubble and into that ward that he lived in. Its a major transition. It can never go back.

And what happens to our baby when it crashes, unknowingly, into every kind of microbe you can imagine? Absolutely nothing. It's usually totally fine. It doesn't even get a temperature. It takes its first breath, is laid on the mother's chest for a hug, and is then covered with a blanket while everybody celebrates.

How Long Does It Take a Baby to Get a Microbiome?

A baby's first contact with microbes is with the ones in the mother's vaginal canal. As it passes through the vagina during the birth process, it then also comes into very close contact with the microbes from the rectum—specifically, the mother's stool microbes. These vaginal and fecal microbes get all over it, over its skin, its nostrils, and its lips. The newborn's ears, in particular, are little microbe scoops, collecting samples on their way through the birth canal. A swab from a newborn's ear can be used instead of a vaginal swab to check for any pathogens in the birth canal.

The new baby's first breath sucks in the microbes of the delivery room air deep into its lungs. The same microbes land in its mouth and are some of the first microbes to be swallowed to enter the gastrointestinal tract. Its next or simultaneous contact is with the microbes on the delivery room surfaces, the blankets, the sheets, and the medical attendant's gloved hands. Thereafter, ideally, the newborn is placed straight onto its mother's chest so that its skin is in contact with its mother's skin, reassuring, and familiar in its smell and warmth and in the sound of the mother's heartbeat. This contact invisibly passes on yet more of the mother's microbes. It's only been seconds since the baby was born, but already it has a microbiome.

But it's not a "proper" microbiome yet. It's simply a diverse set of microbes that have happened to land on the baby's skin. These first microbes are sometimes known as pioneer microbes. They have landed on pure and virgin soil. There is no one else there as yet. But will they stay? Will any survive? (See Figure 4.1.)

If we swab newborn babies in the first minutes, the first hours, and the first days after birth, we see a successive series of pictures. Like snapshots, these document the new arrivals and those first moments of exploration. But these snapshots quickly become more like shots of a battlefield. Microbes are disembarking everywhere; there is mass confusion, and skirmishes and battles are taking place in every direction we look. Not everyone can survive in these territories. Some can only live in oxygen-free conditions, some can't tolerate the dryness; many of them die instantly, some slowly.

The stool bacteria that make it into the mouth and the gut, especially the ones that can cope with oxygen, do well for a while. Known as facultative anaerobes, they can live either with or without oxygen. Eventually they use up the oxygen in the baby's bowel forming a new oxygen-free environment within the baby's gut. This will allow anaerobic bacteria to survive and eventually find a foothold.

66 THE MICROBIOME

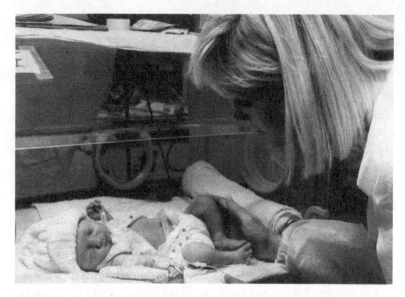

Figure 4.1 This photograph, which depicts a healthcare worker attending to a newborn infant, was used in a public health awareness campaign promoting prenatal care.

The skin bacteria from the mother, the attendant's hands, and those floating around the room can readily cope with the baby's skin habitat if they are lucky enough to land there, being used to the dry, arid nature of skin surfaces. These bacteria may well be able to colonize, especially as babies are no longer washed immediately they are born because of the risk of hypothermia.

The tussle that is going on among these microbes, the struggle to determine which species colonize and which are outcompeted, continues over the first hours and days of the baby's life. Meanwhile, as these battles are being enacted all over its body, the baby is just lying there quite relaxed, sleeping or intermittently feeding.

However, we can see some silent results of this action on the baby in the signs of a condition known as erythema toxicum neonatorum, which causes a transient red rash on the skin. It does not affect all babies, but in about half, it appears for the first few days and causes a blotchy red appearance, especially in areas with hair follicles. Thought to be related to the baby's immune system reacting to new skin microbes, it is common, causes no harm or discomfort, lasts a few days and then goes.

How Do We Know What Is Happening?

Decades of research on newborns and repeated sequential swabs and stool samples have enabled us to work out what is happening to the first microbes that arrive on the baby: when they come, which they are, and which ones stay and colonize. As better scientific techniques have developed over the last century, these experiments have been repeated, each time shedding more light on the processes of neonatal microbiome assembly.

One of the first scientists to study the normal flora of the newborn baby was Theodore Escherich (1857–1911). Escherich was a German pediatrician who started studying medicine in 1876, the exact same year that Koch discovered the microbial cause of anthrax disease. Enabled by the newly established scientific field of bacteriology led by Koch in Berlin, Escherich decided to study the bacteria that could be found in the stools of infants.

He was fully aware that he had chosen a difficult area to study. Each milligram of stool contains literally millions of bacteria and thousands of different types. How was anyone going to be able to differentiate one from another? Almost all were undescribed at this time, and each was of unknown significance. "It would appear to be a pointless and doubtful exercise to examine and disentangle the apparently randomly appearing bacteria in normal faeces and the intestinal tract, a situation that seems controlled by a thousand coincidences."[1]

But Escherich was motivated to study newborn stool because of the high infant mortality he had seen caused by intestinal infections. In Germany during the 1880s, especially in the area of Württemberg near where Escherich was studying in Würzburg, infant mortality was terribly high. At this time, the inhabitants of Württemberg did not believe in breast-feeding their babies, giving them a mixture of flour and water instead. Consequently, infant mortality in this area ran at a devastating 41 percent. Mortality tables by cause, recorded a few decades later in 1910, still show a

68 THE MICROBIOME

similarly high level; of 18,679 deaths in infants under one year of age, over half from gastroenteritis.[2,3]

Escherich, as a city pediatrician, would have been a frequent eyewitness to infant gastroenteritis infections, which, as he said, "still decimate our neonates" and motivated him to try to identify the cause of "this most murderous of all intestinal diseases."

However, because of these high mortality rates, Escherich had access to samples we just don't anymore; he could do autopsies on those newborn babies who had died and see things that we now never see. In a lecture in Munich in 1885, and later in his 1886 groundbreaking work *Enterobacteria of Infants and Their Relation to Digestion Physiology* (*Die Darmbakterien des Säuglings und ihre Beziehungen zur Physiologie der Verdauung*), he starts with a description of the meconium, the initial newborn stool, of two infants who had died during birth and had not yet come into contact with air, which he says, "were sterile as expected."

Does the Baby's Microbiome Change over Time?

Although the meconium starts as sterile, the numbers and types of bacteria rapidly increase, and as Escherich describes, "by 24 hours are demonstrable in large numbers." But this initial collection of microbes changes suddenly and markedly once a milk diet is firmly established. "Instead of the colourful variety of types and forms of the meconium faeces, the bacterial flora now appears to consist of a single type of slender sometimes slightly curved short rods such that a superficial examination might make one assume a pure culture were present."

He carried out ten neonatal autopsies, and in each he describes seeing the milky intestinal contents in the upper part of the intestine and the meconium remaining in the lower parts of the intestine, with the junction or transition from one to the other at variable places, depending on how many days old the infant was when it died. In each case, the upper intestine is already dominated by just one sort of bacteria, but the "colourful variety" of bacteria is still present in the lower part. This shows that this "pure culture of bacteria," of whatever sort it was, was completely dependent on there being the right nutrients and conditions present, in short the breast milk.

He comments on the "remarkable immunity shown by suckling children towards certain infectious diseases," which we will come back to later in the chapter. In addition, he is the first to postulate the key concept of colonization resistance that we met in the previous chapter, noting that "even germs capable of developing under these conditions will have to withstand the struggle for survival with those organisms already present—a struggle that will end with victory for the type most suited to these conditions and total displacement of the other."

When we read his description of the shapes of the different bacteria he sees, though, we really are in the dark about what he is looking at and what the significance of each is. For example, he describes the "little-head bacterium": "Not unlike a spermatozoon in shape, and at the end of a 4−7 micrometre long slender stalk it carries a bright, glittering spore." It is not possible to identify from these descriptions which microbe he is referring to.

Escherich was groundbreaking in his neonatal research and yet necessarily limited in his conclusions. He must have been seeing and describing what we now know are anaerobic bacteria in this almost "pure culture" of milk-fed stools, but he did not have the techniques to culture them or characterize them further. Instead, he sensibly focused on the bacteria that he could culture and managed to securely identify a small rod-shaped bacterium, which he called *Bacterium coli commune*.

Because of its shape, he assumed that this bacterium was that same predominant organism that he had observed in a milk-fed baby's stools.[4] Although he was wrong about the significance of *Bacterium coli commune* in this context, this rod-shaped bacterium was a key discovery, highly prevalent in the human gut, certainly present in the infant gut, and possibly one of the most studied bacteria known today. It was later renamed *Escherichia coli* in his honor.[5]

Which Bacteria Are in a Baby's Microbiome?

Escherich's work on studying the intestinal flora of newborn babies was taken forward by many other scientists. In 1899, a scientist named Henri Tissier finally managed to isolate and culture the microbe dominating milk-fed baby's stools that Escherich had observed, naming it *Bacillus bifidus communis*. Now referred to as *Bifidobacterium longum*, this key species accounts for over 99 percent of bacteria in a breastfed infant's stool.

Taking advantage of new developments in aerobic and anaerobic culture methods, two scientists, Ivan C. Hall and Elizabeth O'Toole, working in Denver, Colorado, repeated the observations in 1929 on fifty newborn infants. They identified eighteen different species, including *Bifidobacterium longum* and *Escherichia coli*, but also *Lactobacillus acidophilus*, another key lactose-fermenting microbe, and other bacteria such as *Streptococcus faecalis*, now called *Enterococcus faecalis*, and *Hay bacillus*, a name that has fallen out of use entirely but probably refers to *Bacillus subtilis*.[6]

Hall and O'Toole summarize the current thinking of the time, still in line with Escherich's findings: "We know that the meconium is generally sterile at birth, that various bacteria appear in it within the first twenty-four hours of life, that the flora of the first three or four days is complex, that simplification accompanies the establishment of normal lactation . . . that diversification in the flora . . . normally follows weaning . . . and that even in the adult a preponderance of lactose, in milk . . . may again bring about a simplification of the intestinal flora in the direction of that shown by a healthy nursing infant."

Research on the developing flora of newborns has continued over the following decades, accounting for hundreds of studies. More recently, genetic techniques, instead of culture-based techniques, have enabled "deeper dives" into neonatal stool bacterial diversity but marry well with earlier studies. Everywhere from Sweden to Japan describes that initial heady mix of aerobic or facultative anaerobes, such as enterobacteria, enterococci, and staphylococci, followed by later domination by various acid-producing bacteria, most especially the bifidobacteria species, including *Bifidobacterium longum*, *Bifidobacterium breve*, *Bifidobacterium adolescentis*, and

Bifidobacterium bifidum. Eventually, a ratio of 1,000 bifidobacteria is established for every 1 enterobacterium in infant stool.[7]

Do Babies Get Their Bacteria from the Mother's Vagina?

Studies obtaining samples from newborns and their mothers—so-called mother-baby dyads—offer even more information, not just on which bacteria are in neonatal stool but on where they come from.

Metagenomic studies, such as the "Mother-to-Infant" trial, have specifically focused on this by examining mother-baby dyad samples to strain-level detail. Taking samples from the baby's tongue and stool and the mother's tongue, skin, stool, and vagina, at frequent time intervals—birth, day one, day three, one week, one month, and four months—it gives us a sequential view, an almost filmic idea, of which bacteria are there at which time and which ones make it through from the initial transfer at birth to be present four months later.[8]

This study identified not just eighteen species in newborn stools as in 1925. It picked up a further 369 genomes, some representing bacteria yet to be described. It is clear from these samples that each baby's initial mix depends on which bacteria it has happened to bump into in its first hours—usually vaginal, stool, or skin-based species. Because of this random element, each baby's stools are initially completely different from any others. This initial variation is much reduced by day seven, with a "simplification" of the intestinal microbiome as it starts to lean toward bifidobacteria and increased similarity between babies.

It has been assumed in the past that because the baby exits the womb via the vaginal passage that it is the mother's vaginal bacteria that colonize the baby and the vaginal bacteria that it needs. Some practitioners have even suggested that babies who have missed out on picking up bacteria from the birth canal because of a caesarean birth should be given a bacterial top-up, by wiping a flannel over the mother's genitals and then over the baby's face.

But the "Mother-to-Infant" study shows that vaginal bacteria have only a transient moment in the sun. They are certainly present to start with. Easily detected on initial skin and stool samples, they land in large numbers on the baby's ears, eyes, face, and skin. But they don't make it. Swabs from the baby a few days later fail to pick up any vaginal bacteria at all.

Some scientists describe this disappearance of a pioneer species as the baby "curating" the bacteria. Curating is a nice idea and seems to suggest that the baby deliberately decides which bacteria it keeps and which it doesn't. But the presence of any one bacterium is a simple matter of survival. The lactic bacteria of the vagina, like every species, need a specific environmental niche to survive. But they don't find this niche on the new baby anywhere, neither in its mouth, its gut, or in any crevice. They simply die, killed by other nearby bacteria or dispatched by the baby's immune system and shed by its barrier systems. We can't see the deaths in our swab and sample snapshots; all we see is their absence.

So, which bacteria do survive on the baby if it is not the vaginal bacteria? The pioneers most likely to survive are the stool bacteria. Not many people will want to imagine that that perfect newborn baby they are holding (with that special newborn smell) has especially been colonized by bacteria obtained from stool. But that is what we have to get our heads around.

And not just any stool bacteria from random passersby, the environment, or even the father. When analyzed to strain-specific detail, the best survivors on the newborn baby are the *mother's* stool bacteria. Each mother's personal stool bacteria account for over 40 percent of the microbial population present in the first few days of the baby's life and 22 percent of the species. They are also the most likely ones to successfully colonize and still be present four months later, typically accounting for 60 percent of the overall gut microbial population at this time. Whether being an early arrival gives these bacteria a survival advantage, or the genetic connection between the mother and the baby means her particular strains are more likely to survive, or whether their survival is simply a matter of chance, is simply not known.

Where Do Babies Born by Caesarean Get Their Bacteria From?

What about babies born by caesarean? They do not run the gamut through the vagina and past the mother's perineal area. They are taken out of the mother through a sterile abdominal incision and into the clean conditions of the theater. Does that mean they stay clean? And does it give them an advantage or a disadvantage over vaginally born babies?

Babies born by caesarean section, although born into a very clean room, are not born into a sterile room. However sterile the surgical drapes and the gloved hands of the medical staff are, the air is not sterile. At the moment of birth, the caesarean-born baby enters our microbial world like any other, and its first breath is just like that of a vaginally born baby—a large, deep breath of microbial-infested air, some of which they swallow.

Briefly thereafter, their experience is a little different. The first skin contact for a caesarean-born baby is not with the bacteria on the warm surface of its mother's genitals, but with the rather impersonal collection of bacteria from the operating theater dust. Studies have shown, by swabbing the floors, walls, ventilation grids, and armrests of the C-section room, but most especially the tops of surgical lamps, that the "clean" surfaces in a surgical theater yield plenty of bacteria, mostly human skin ones such as *Staphylococcus* and *Corynebacterium*.[9]

Swabs prove that a caesarean-born baby starts life with a different amount and set of bacteria from a baby born vaginally. So, will a caesarean baby's health be affected by that brief divergence from the usual path of being born and dosed by millions of bacteria?

Does Missing Out on Bacteria at Birth Cause Future Health Problems?

The difference in health between babies born vaginally and those born by caesarean section is a subject that has been studied extensively. Many health outcomes have been measured, from counting the number of chest infections the caesarean-born experience as children, to their rates of heart disease and diabetes when they are fifty. When all the data is summed up, there is a proven difference. A meta-analysis combining a large number of studies (n=887,960) demonstrates a link between being born by caesarean section and, specifically, the development of childhood asthma (odds ratio (OR) 1.2) and obesity (OR 1.6).[10]

It is a significant leap to assume that this increase in asthma and obesity is because those individuals came across the wrong sort or the wrong amount of bacteria during their first moments of life. However, the "hygiene hypothesis"—the idea that living in an environment that is too clean leads to allergies—may be relevant here. There are several significant ongoing studies that are looking at the link between microbe exposure and allergy development, and we will come back to this important topic in the last chapter, on microbiome diversity.

Does the difference in microbe exposure last? Although the caesarean-born baby has avoided a large dose of vaginal and stool bacteria for the time being, if it is given to the mother to hold, with skin-to-skin contact and a towel to keep it warm, just like a vaginally born baby, their experiences start to converge again. Some studies show there is no significant difference in the microbiome between the vaginally born and the caesarean born by the six-week mark.[11]

This is because the transfer of bacteria from the mother does not just take place at birth; it happens continuously. There are countless chances for the mother to transfer microbes to the newborn every time it feeds and with every contact it has with the mother. And the mother's stool bacteria don't account for all of the bacteria living it up in their new home; the baby is constantly being "seeded" by contacts it makes with the rest of its family too. Both parents are likely to be heavy donors (and will typically have somewhat of a shared microbiome with each other anyway), but the baby's siblings, its environment, or even its pets will all contribute. No matter how the baby is born, it will have plenty of opportunities to come into contact with plenty of bacteria.

How Do Anaerobic Bacteria Survive the Transfer?

We can imagine that some bacteria easily manage the transfer from mother to baby, but how do the strict stool anaerobes make it when they are so sensitive to the toxic effects of oxygen? That they do is obvious, and that they have a cunning plan to transfer to the next generation every time by living so close to the birth canal. It is clear from the strain-level analysis on mother-infant dyads that birth is the main moment of transmission. But how? Can they somehow hold their breath?

Many bacteria have developed strategies to survive outside of their preferred environments. One of these is to form into a spore (or more specifically an endospore) rather than forming two new bacteria when they divide. Like tiny, tough little seeds, endospores can survive dry, energy-poor conditions indefinitely before germinating and replicating again—and using this method of survival can easily effect a transfer from mother to baby. An alternative method of survival for non-sporulating bacteria is known as dormancy, in which the cell walls are altered and metabolism slows, enabling survival in harsh conditions. But for those microbes without either the option of sporulation or dormancy, transfer can be more precarious.

Tests have shown that some strict anaerobes can survive for up to six hours in exposure to the air, so there is leeway for them to survive the transfer—especially if they have the good luck to land on or near the mouth or get quickly under cover. The alternative explanation is to consider the microenvironment. Maybe the transfer is enabled inside a small particle, perhaps sealing up a tiny anaerobic chamber with the anaerobic bacteria inside, or maybe the transfer succeeds by closely covering up the anaerobic bacteria with organic matter in some way.

Metagenomic techniques can specifically track the journey of anaerobic bacteria in more detail than has been possible before and show that these species are present from the first day, already accounting for almost one-sixth of the bacteria present, even at this early stage. By day three, their numbers have drastically decreased. But, as the life-threatening oxygen levels in the infant gut begins to decrease, the anaerobes gain confidence, and by day seven, their numbers are on the up again.

Are Newborn Babies Born Sterile?

It has been assumed since the beginning of the study of microbiology that unborn babies still in the womb are sterile. But to everyone's surprise, in 2014 scientists published a study claiming that samples of placenta taken from inside the uterus had detectable bacterial DNA present. These

76 THE MICROBIOME

unexpected results led some scientists to announce the presence of an intrauterine microbiome, reopening the 150-year debate on the sterility of the womb.

The idea that babies could be born with a microbiome ready formed, rather than picking one up via the birth canal, was seismic news. The story was seized upon by the press soon after the paper was published, perhaps without the journalists quite realizing what a significant announcement it was. For microbes to be found in a part of the body long known to be sterile, was not just vaguely interesting or even groundbreaking research. It was earth-shattering news—equivalent to CERN announcing that light is actually not a wave at all or that evolution is not a thing.

But long-held theories can be overturned in science. If all the evidence adds up and the experiments can be replicated, then the world sometimes simply has to accept a new theory of everything. The researchers working on the metagenomics of the uterus must have been thrilled to be in at the start of something so massive.

Their evidence was straightforward: 16S rRNA and whole-genome shotgun analysis on samples from 320 placental samples collected under sterile conditions had picked up genomes consistent with bacteria. "In aggregate, the placental microbiome profiles were most akin to the human oral microbiome."[12]

Medical microbiology consultants were baffled. If it were true that the uterus had its own microbiome that in turn seeded the fetus, it would overturn everything they had ever been taught. Nothing they had understood during an entire career would make sense anymore.

For a practicing clinical doctor though, working with actual patients every day, this announcement would at best seem highly unlikely. Women cannot have bacteria in utero. They would just die—as everybody knows. If during labor the amniotic fluid begins to leak out of the vagina it is said that "the waters have broken" because the seal to the uterine sac has literally broken. The cervical plug has come away, and there is now a small hole in the amniotic membrane. That's why the fluids surrounding the baby leak out. Usually, the woman then goes into labor immediately. But if she does not, she is watched over very carefully. If any raised temperature is detected, labor is induced immediately. Because now the amniotic sac has been breached, bacteria can enter and cause a serious infection. The longer the pregnant woman is left untreated, the more likely it is that she will get a fever, develop sepsis, and that she and the baby become very ill, or even die, from a uterine infection. Bacteria in utero is not a joke. It's a life-or-death situation.

But the more microbiome specialists discussed this issue, the more they came up with strange and implausible ideas. For example, the "maternal gut-utero axis," in which they postulated that bacteria could travel from the mother's gut into the bloodstream and from there through the placenta to the baby.[13] Of course, we know that maternal antibodies and other immune molecules cross the placenta, protecting the newborn for the first two to three months of its life. But actual bacteria do not travel through the maternal bloodstream to reach the baby's bloodstream unless the mother has bacteremia, which usually implies severe sepsis.

How Reliable Is Microbiome Research When Studying "Low or No Biomass" Areas of the Body?

The short answer is, not very reliable. The difficulty with metagenomics is that it is almost too sensitive. No matter what you test with it, and however careful you are to get a sterile sample, it will pick up some genomic material somewhere. When dealing with a high biomass sample such as stool, the genetic material from the bacteria is so rich that any "white noise" from the technique is irrelevant. But in a low biomass sample from, say, a sterile surface, the test will pick up genetic material no matter what—very small amounts of it: genetic material that has floated in from the air, that has dropped in from the technician's hands, and even material that is already present in the testing equipment, on the labware, tools, instruments, on reagents, and in DNA isolation kits, the so-called "kitome." It is not unreasonable to ask, is this is even the right test for studying sterile areas? Would it actually be possible to prove that an area is sterile using metagenomics?

Many microbiome specialists did not get involved in the prenatal microbiome debate, attributing the controversy to a misguided "vocal minority."

78 THE MICROBIOME

But research papers working on the topic couldn't ignore it and had to mention the issue in some way, even if they thought it wrong. For example, "The role and importance of prenatal microbial colonization are still open to debate" (see note 8). This is a reasonably neat way of sidestepping the issue, but it perpetuates the error. Papers often quote each other, and when the topic enters textbooks and even trusted resources like Wikipedia: "The human infant gut is relatively sterile up until birth," you know it's game over, and this misinformation is going to be hard to claw back.

But metagenomics does not work out scientific theories in isolation from other scientific techniques, nor should microbiome specialists work on the microbiome in isolation from other specialists. The authors of "A Philosophical Perspective on the Prenatal In Utero Microbiome Debate" were integral to establishing a transdisciplinary group of scientists aimed at resolving the issue. This group included not only microbiome specialists but also clinicians, obstetricians, bioinformatics specialists, immunologists, microbiologists, and scientists who specialize in germ-free animals.[14]

One of the most imaginative studies analyzed during this collaboration was one that, like many others, tested the first-pass meconium of twenty babies. But not just any babies. These babies had to be known breech babies (babies being born bottom first) and, as well, booked for a caesarean. In the sterile environment of the surgical theater—wearing the full kit of gloves, gowns, hats, and masks—the researchers inserted a swab straight through the surgical caesarean incision and into the baby's anus -with the baby still completely inside the mother. In this way, they obtained a sample of the ultimate first-pass meconium.

Not content with this jaw-droppingly rigorous methodology, they also took a comprehensive series of controls and blank samples, from the theater, the lab, and at every stage of the analysis to allow measurement of DNA contamination.

Of course, they still picked up bacterial genetic material in over 50 percent of samples, but these matched either the genera typical of the kitome, such as *Halomonas* and *Rhodanobacter*, or bacteria commonly found on environmental surfaces, such as *Staphylococcus epidermidis* (a skin bacterium) or *Micrococcus* (a typical contaminant found in water, dust, and soil).

They concluded firmly, as per the title of their paper: "Fetal meconium does not have a detectable microbiota before birth."[15]

The transdisciplinary group analyzed a wide range of contradictory papers from the perspective of each specialty. Bioinformatics specialists reported back on the "misapplication of contamination removal programs like decontam," which are computer-based algorithms designed to "clean the data" of contaminants by simply deleting some of the DNA code thought to be inaccurate. Microbiologists noted biologically implausible taxa reported as present in placental tissues, such as *Gloeobacter*, a photosynthetic cyanobacterium more typical of the ocean.

From an immunological standpoint, it was observed that if there were a uterine microbiome, there would have to be a mechanism by which the fetus could first tolerate bacterial populations and second avoid inflammation and tissue destruction (i.e., death). No such immunological mechanism has been proposed, let alone identified.

Lastly, the germ-free animal evidence was particularly obvious; if there were microbes in utero, how would scientists have been able to sustain microbe-free animal colonies for so many decades?

Taken together, the evidence does not support "stable abundant colonizers in the healthy human fetus." This phrase allows for the fact that bacteria sometimes do get into the uterus accidentally (and cause infection), but emphasizes that this accidental infiltration is different from an established and consistent microbiome.[16]

The sterile uterus debate may seem like a small storm in a test tube, only interesting to microbiome specialists or to those actually studying neonates. But the uterine environment being sterile is fundamental to the whole of medicine and microbiology, and the deeply misleading statements on this topic in research papers and textbooks need to be updated and revised. As the transdisciplinary group points out, mistakes like this have significant costs, not least the monetary one. "Tens of millions of dollars have been spent to investigate microbial populations that likely do not exist."

There are lessons to be learned here. About the use of metagenomics for "low- or no-biomass research," which is still continuing fruitlessly in other areas known to be sterile, such as the brain, blood, and cancer tumors.

80 THE MICROBIOME

About the sidelining of decades of accumulated scientific evidence on the sterile womb debate. And about the importance of collaboration with other scientific specialties. It is hoped that the principles established here will be applied appropriately in the future to avoid both the further waste of resources and the misdirection.

How Does the Baby Survive in a Microbial World?

We have said that the baby is relaxed and tolerates meeting thousands of pioneer microbes quietly and without any outward effect on its health. But we have also said how vulnerable newborns are and talked about how many of the newborns that Escherich would have seen did not survive their first year. How do we explain these contradictions?

The difference in survival is partly a matter of which bacteria the baby comes across first. Most of the bacteria in our environment are not pathogens. They are mostly not invasive and do not have additional extra endangering abilities such as toxin production. There is no innate way of telling a pathogen from another bacteria; indeed, as we have already seen, some bacteria can swap roles depending on their circumstances. But we do have lists of human pathogens that have been identified one by one according to documented human infections, and these lists suggest that pathogens account for just 7 percent of all validly described bacterial species (1,513 pathogens in total).[17]

We don't want the baby to meet the fast-acting aggressive pathogens first (or indeed ever, but we can't guarantee that); we want them to meet the ordinary bacteria first. This is because the baby's immune system needs time to get activated. The immune system is primed for action at birth, ready to be set off as soon as it meets its first bacteria, just like in our germ-free animals. The lymph nodes are all present, the Peyer's patches are there in the gut, and the Paneth cells are in the intestinal crypts ready to secrete antimicrobial compounds. But at this stage, the lymph nodes and groups of immune cells are small, reflecting the fact that they are still quiescent. They are waiting for their first meeting with . . . they don't know what.

But when the innate immune system meets its first bacteria, it knows. Parts of the bacterial cell wall are only ever found on bacteria and are chemically distinct from every other living creature. The attacking cells of the innate immune system are primed to recognize these bacterial cell wall components and by this automatically recognize bacteria -no matter what sort. They do not differentiate between pathogens and other bacteria; they dispose of them all.

But it takes time for the innate immune system cell processes to move. The macrophages have to travel through the tissues. The cytotoxins must diffuse, and the B-cells and T-cells of the adaptive immune system have to be presented with their first antigen before they can be activated. It is better if the innate immune system is activated by a relatively benign bacterium first.

Within hours of bacteria hitting the gut, the Peyer's patches and lymph nodes begin to enlarge, the mucosa begins to thicken, the crypts become deeper, and the villi broader and shorter, and, overall, the mass of the small intestine increases. The genes regulating intestinal epithelial cell turnover and mucous biosynthesis are turned on, and a thick layer of intestinal mucous is produced to protect the cells of the gut lining. Antimicrobial compounds begin to be secreted from Paneth cells, and in addition to this, intestinal peristalsis suddenly increases. Like switching on the down escalator in a theater to evacuate people after a terrific show and get them out of the building, the rippling action of the peristalsis in the gut constantly moves the bacteria out of the gut.[18]

Together, all of these activities protect the newborn. They improve the gut barrier function, reduce the overall number of bacteria in the gut and increase the newborn's chances of eliminating any bacteria present in the wrong place. Some people describe all these activities as a function of the microbiome, that the microbiome activates the baby's immune system. But is it fair to call this a "function" of the fetal microbiome? It is obvious that the newborn baby wouldn't have to activate its immune system if it didn't have to cope with its microbiome.

Taken together, when we think about these immune strategies and barrier functions in the newborn, all triggered by the baby's first encounters

82 THE MICROBIOME

with microbes, it's almost as if the newborn doesn't want any "friendly" bacteria in its gut. In a similar way to the skin's innate defenses, it appears to be using every strategy possible to reduce or eliminate bacteria. But of course, just like the skin, it can't keep the gut sterile. It can't have sterility as its goal; that would not be practical. The newborn must somehow manage the constant stream of new bacteria entering its body. But are any of the bacteria wanted? Are any of them actually "friendly"?

Does the Fetal Microbiome Cause Problems for the Newborn?

It's hard to work out and prove what any one bacterium, let alone a group of bacteria, might possibly do for us. But what is clear is that the impact of all of these bacteria landing on the gut is a strain for the newborn in its first few weeks of its life and causes a marked inflammation of the gut.

We know this because we can measure gut inflammation using a test called fecal calprotectin. A high level of fecal calprotectin reflects a high level of mucosal inflammation in the gut. It's a very effective test, often used in patients with inflammatory bowel disease, and has revolutionized the management of conditions such as Crohn's disease and ulcerative colitis.

In adults, a normal reading is less than 60 micrograms per milligram, but a typical reading for a neonate is 100 to 300. The readings are not easy to interpret in the neonate because calprotectin is also found in breast milk, but when controlled for this the readings in neonates are still high and reflect the activity going on in the gut to defend against bacteria, as well as the resulting inflammation.

We have said that babies quietly sleep and feed while major revolutions in their microbiomes are going on. But as babies get a little older, many of them do start to cry more, and some of them appear to suffer from tummy aches. Abdominal pain and crying in a baby is often known as colic, a nonspecific condition difficult to define. But if an otherwise healthy baby is crying for more than three hours a day, more than three days a week, for more than one week, it can be diagnosed as having colic. Up to one-fifth of babies are thought to get it, peaking at six weeks but settling by four months.

In babies with colic, fecal calprotectin levels are even higher, between 600 and 700 micrograms per milligram.[19] This gives us a new understanding of the discomfort they must be experiencing. Comparisons of the stool microbiome in babies with colic compared to those without suggest that the condition may be caused by an imbalance of the baby's gut microbiome, perhaps due to a lack of bifidobacteria or alternatively to an overgrowth of *Acinetobacter* spp.[20]

What Are Bifidobacteria?

We have talked a lot about bifidobacteria: that to start with babies don't have them, and then they have lots; that they might be important for the baby's health; and that a lack of them may be associated with colic. We know they are hardly visible at all at birth but that they bloom once milk feeds are established. We also know that bifidobacteria are well conserved across species. Many newborn animals, including primates, rats, mice, and rabbits, have their own versions of bifidobacteria spp. in the stool of their milk-fed young.[21]

This consistent dominance of just one sort of microbe in the intestines of babies across the world and across animal species, means that the microbiome of the newborn gut is completely different from the other microbiomes we have mentioned so far. It is marked not by a huge variety but a huge uniformity, implying that this bacterium is important to our health. So what are these bacteria?

In the words of Cruickshank, an early researcher on bifidobacteria writing in 1925, bifidobacteria are "rather slender, straight or slightly curved Gram-positive bacillus of variable length—from 2 to 7 micrometres although the majority are 4–5 micrometres in length, and about 0.7 micrometres in breadth. The extremities are rather round and often at one or both ends is a bulbous thickening." The "bifido" in the name refers to the tendency of bifidobacteria to sometimes form bifurcated or Y-shaped forms.[22] They are non-motile and do not move around or invade the baby's tissues, nor do they spore. Their optimum growth temperature is 37 degrees centigrade, close to the core temperature of

84   THE MICROBIOME

a neonate, and they have the advantage of being able to grow over a wide pH range, from 4.0 to 7.0. It may be that this acid tolerance of bifidobacteria may be their most important quality with respect to the neonate.

When the baby starts to obtain breast milk, the milk has a pH of 6.35, but this soon drops as the lactic acid bacteria in the baby's gut start to metabolize the nutrients in the milk. The lactose, a milk sugar, is fermented by bifidobacteria and other acid-tolerant bacteria, which digest the lactose to form lactic acid, carbon dioxide, and hydrogen. The acid reduces the pH of infant stool to between 4.8 and 5.0, a level that stops most other bacteria growing and reduces the overall number of bacterial species. This suits the baby very well as it reduces the chance of a gastroenteritis infection, and it also suits the bifidobacteria, which then do not have to compete with other bacteria for resources.

Although bifidobacteria don't like acid conditions that much, they tolerate it much better than other bacteria, which gives them the edge for survival. Bifidobacteria colonization of the neonatal gut must be helping to protect the baby from gastrointestinal infections and is another important example of colonization protection. As Cruickshank explains, "The presence of an almost purely aciduric flora, together with the high degree of acidity in the breast-fed infant's intestine, acts as a protective agent, particularly against invasion by organisms of the coli group, and this may explain in part at least the relative immunity of the breast-fed child to gastro-enteritis" (see note 22).

Bifidobacteria are mainly dependent on milk as their nutrient substrate and will appear in great numbers, almost magically, if there is a milk diet. A study conducted in 1915 on adult rats fed a diet consisting solely of milk showed that within days, animals that initially had no detectable bifidobacteria at all had stools dominated by bifidobacteria. These bacteria disappeared again when milk feeding was discontinued.[23]

As well as metabolizing lactose, some scientists believe that bifidobacteria utilize another important element within the milk known as human milk oligosaccharides (HMOs).[24] It is thought that HMOs are processed by bifidobacteria, producing metabolites which can be utilized by the baby as an energy source, giving it a small growth advantage of about 1 to 2 percent.[25] However, it is not absolutely certain that this is the case.[26]

Indeed, the importance of HMOs might be better explained by their antimicrobial action. HMOs have an anti-adhesive effect on pathogens which stops them causing bacterial infections. The large variety of HMOs (over 200 different types) is an advantage, as each version can protect against a different microbe.[27]

There is no doubt that the presence of bifidobacteria is desirable in that it indicates a healthy breastfed infant. But is it simply an indicator? A surrogate measurement for health rather than healthy in itself? Some breastfed infants do not have a predominance of bifidobacteria, and others have no bifidobacteria at all, yet they thrive. Other infants are unable to breastfeed and thrive well on formula milk with or without bifidobacteria.[28] However, the acidic environment of the stool that is engendered by bifidobacteria does appear to be an important strategy to prevent unwanted pathogens from colonizing and overall must improve the survival chances of a human infant.

If we want to improve the health of an infant then, should we be encouraging skin-to-skin contact, or should we be washing the baby thoroughly after birth? And should we be giving them breast milk, supplementing them with HMOs to help fight off infection, supplementing them with HMOs to help feed their bifidobacteria or administering bifidobacteria probiotics?

Breastfeeding is one of the keys to good infant health, and this is reflected in the World Health Organization's (WHO) advice, in a way bypassing microbiome research. WHO does not recommend probiotics, bifidobacteria, or HMO supplementation. It simply advises all new mothers to breastfeed their babies based on large, well-run studies that prove the protective effect of breastfeeding against gastrointestinal infections. This advice supports what Escherich and others have known for generations: that breastfeeding helps newborn infants survive.[29]

If only Escherich's patients had believed in breastfeeding instead of feeding their infants flour mixed with water, then maybe these babies would have survived too.

5

THE MICROBIOME AND THE GUT

The gut microbiome is, of course, the key microbiome of the human body. This is the microbiome we are most familiar with and the one most discussed. If we talk about the microbiome, it will most likely be about the gut microbes and if someone has not heard the word microbiome, "the friendly bacteria in our intestines" is a good shorthand way of explaining, and a familiar notion to many.

The subject of intestinal health is intensely interesting to many people, not just people with infections or serious illnesses. We are all making decisions about what to eat on a daily basis, and we feel the natural consequences of those decisions—whether the food has made us feel full or left us hungry, and whether we are fine over the next few hours or have experienced stomach aches and bloating. For most of us, monitoring these sorts of eating experiences is a daily experiment that never loses its interest.

What, then, if we could monitor this in even more detail and consider not just the taste or the calories of the food but also the microbes that come with it?

Should I Get a Gut Test to Check My Microbes?

To monitor our gut microbiome in detail, it might at first glance seem sensible to get a gut microbiome test. We could have a range of gut microbes checked for between $200 and $300. Many options are available, and each testing company has a different combination of tests a available. It can be confusing trying to choose between a "gut intelligence test," an "essential gut health test," or an "ultimate test," but a typical high end option might include tests that check both a set of medical parameters and a collection of more novel gut microbe tests, to get a sense of our own personal microbiome. The more conventional medical tests can include analyzing the stool for traces of blood and inflammatory markers to check for gut inflammation, or checking for the presence of well-known pathogens such as giardia, salmonella, or norovirus. In contrast, the more novel gut microbial tests will culture a set of microbes that are usually part of the gut microbiome. This will typically include a list of at least twenty different bacteria and fungi, such as *Bacteroides* spp., *Bifidobacterium* spp., *Lactobacillus* spp., *Clostridium* spp., *Corynebacterium* spp., *Enterococcus* spp., *Candida albicans*, and a few others. They often also give a sense of the prevalence of each; +++ if there are a lot, + if only a few.

The more conventional medical tests, the blood in the stool, the inflammatory markers are easy to interpret. We are used to analyzing these tests in the medical world and know what is normal and what is not. It is the microbiome check that is hard to make sense of. This is because a key finding of the human gut microbiome is its immense variability. Because the gut microbes are different for each person it means we just don't know what a normal result looks like.

But although hard to interpret, commercial stool analyses like these are still a good starting point for visualizing the complexity of the gut microbiome. The bacteria and yeasts it has picked up give us a sense of the different sorts of microbes typically found in a normal stool, and the pathogens it has not picked up give us an idea of what should not be present.

The answer to the question, "Should I get a gut test to check my microbes?" is yes, for a bit of fun, if you want to and can afford it. But if you ever get gastrointestinal symptoms that you are actually worried about, you should speak to your doctor and get a proper assessment. Don't rely on an online microbiome stool test.

88 THE MICROBIOME

What Does the Intestinal Tract Look Like from the Inside?

A stool analysis such as a commercial microbiome analysis described above gives us a window to the end part of the bowel, because it is based on the stool. But this is not enough to work out what is properly going on in the gut, as it only represents one location: the rectum. At best, it is only a surrogate for what is actually going on in this location. Stool samples are easy to obtain and convenient to test, but at the end of the day, an analysis of our stool is more like a summary of what might be happening inside us rather than a detailed analysis. This is because our intestine is not the same all the way along; we don't find stool in our stomach or stomach acids in our colon. Similarly, the microbes we find at one end are a lot different from those we find at the other. To properly find out what is happening inside us, we need to look with a little more magnification and focus.

If we look inside the abdominal cavity (and many of us may have seen surgical procedures on television lit up by surgical spotlights), we see intensely bright colors. The intestines are a glossy baby-pink color and move spontaneously in response to peristalsis, the automatic rippling action of the bowel. The fat attached to the edges of the intestines is a bright butter-yellow, the connective tissue a dazzling, clean white, and any blood is crimson red like geranium petals. But a surgical incision into the abdominal cavity is in the clean zone, and we don't want the clean zone. We want to look where the microbes are—inside the intestines. Here, we will see a much dimmer, more shadowy place.

To visualize the inside of the intestines, we will need to remember every kind of tunnel, cave, or channel we have ever been inside of, starting with the nearest activity swimming pool and those water chutes we never particularly want to go down (but enjoy once we're on).

That dim, diffuse light and that narrow, enclosed feeling of being inside a chute that we experience as we kick off at the start of the ride, is a good approximation for the start of the gastrointestinal tract. The water swishing us rapidly down and the splash into the first pool are as if we are a mouthful of food just swallowed, being washed down the gullet with saliva and landing in a pool of gastric acid in the stomach. If we were really taking this journey, we would need a good light source as well as an excellent protective suit, to protect us from the different digestive juices that we will meet.

The water chute that exits us from the stomach pool marks the start of the small intestine. It goes a little slower, but not much. There is still plenty of liquid swishing us along, and there are still plenty of twists and turns to experience. A sudden steep turn past the liver and gallbladder and we are unexpectedly squirted with a jet of bright yellow bile from a tiny opening right at eye level (we adjust our goggles). Moments later, there is another squirt of some sort of transparent fluid, which turns out to be a stream of deadly protease—protein-digesting enzymes excreted from the pancreas. This section of the chute still looks pink but is much shinier and slipperier than before. It seems to be covered all over with a clear, firm mucus. If we try to slow down the ride by grabbing the internal surface, we find we can't actually touch the walls at all unless we really press into this stuff.

As we slide on, we can see that the surface of this part of the chute has become wrinkled and that the wrinkles overlap each other in places. Within each wrinkle is an undulating surface, and on this surface are hundreds of tiny little villi—little finger-like projections that make up the delightfully named brush border. Villi, undulations, wrinkles, and overlaps all add up to a massive surface area to help absorption of the nutritious liquids that are pouring down with us; typically, 2 liters of intestinal fluids are washed through with every meal.

After several hours of further twists and turns, the ride becomes slower and slower, a bit like one of those fairground rides that feel like they are never going to end (in fact, your journey through the small intestine lasts about eighteen hours). We exit at last into the final channel: the large intestine. This section is much more cavernous and slow, more like a large sewage pipe than a chute, and the pace is now completely different. Instead of sliding, we walk along the edge, easily keeping up with the pace of the liquid as it moves through.

Again, we notice clear mucus all over the surface of the channel. This time, when we try to push our hand into it, it seems to be in two layers, the surface mucus flowing along over a much stiffer mucus underneath. It's more or less impossible to push through it; it resists our pressing, as if we

90 THE MICROBIOME

are being kept at a distance. It prevents us from touching the epithelial cell surface.

If we look above our heads but without touching, we can just make out tiny goblet cells scattered among the epithelial cells, visible through the distorting mucus layers. The goblet cells are the cells that actually make the mucus and it both fills them and is attached to them, making it a difficult-to-remove layer. The epithelial cells are completely replaced every two to five days, but the mucus is replaced at an even faster rate, with a complete changeover occurring every one to two hours.[1]

If we now look down at the sewage-like material in the middle of the channel, we can see it is quite watery. The main function of the large intestine is to absorb water and salts, and we can see the liquid gradually being removed, leaving a more stool-like substance ready for excretion.

Now that we have had a good look and seen the environment of the gut changing all the way down, we can see exactly why a stool analysis represents, at most, a brief summary of what is going on in the gut. In fact, you could argue that a stool analysis gives a better understanding of the microbial activity of the stool than it does of the colon.[2] If we really wanted to get a sense of the microbiome of the gut, we would need to take samples at every stage of the journey and from every surface: the epithelial cell surface, the inner mucus, the outer mucus, and the material in the lumen. We can be sure that each would give us a different reading. Biopsies of the various layers would be even better, and staining would reveal the location of bacteria in the microarchitecture.

When samples from the esophagus, stomach, and small intestine are analyzed, they contain a relatively low yield of bacteria—about 100 colony-forming units (CFU) per milliliter in the stomach and 1,000 CFU per milliliter in the small intestine. The intestinal barrier systems that we have just witnessed on our journey through the intestine, the speed of the transit (driven by peristalsis, not just gravity), the large volumes of liquid, the lethal pool of gastric acid in the stomach, the bile, the pancreatic juice, and the massive surface area of villi allowing the rapid absorption of nutrients (reducing the nutrients available for the bacteria), along with the frequent shedding of the epithelial cells that line the gut and the rapid replacement of the mucus, all combine to reduce bacterial numbers in the small intestine, just as the barrier systems and innate defense systems do for the skin—if not by killing them outright, then by moving them through.

It is not until we reach the large intestine that things get interesting from a microbiome perspective (see Figure 5.1). It is here, that the flow is deliberately slowed, and the channel widens. This material is here for sixty to seventy hours, much longer than we usually imagine, allowing the bacteria time to multiply, reaching the astounding level of 1,000 trillion bacteria per milliliter, contrasting nicely with the 100−1,000 bacteria per milliliter seen in the stomach and small intestine.

By the time the material in the large intestine has been fully processed and formed into a stool ready for excretion, it weighs about 400 grams, consisting partly of water, of course, and partly of shed epithelial cells and undigested fiber. But the remaining 50 percent is made up of bacteria—a third of them dead, a third of them injured, and a third of them viable.

Which Microbes Are in the Gut?

It must be said that trying to work out which microbes are present in the gut has a curiously elusive quality, let alone figuring out how many of each there are or what they actually do. However we try to fix on the correct ones, the list appears to slide out of view, and no matter what we do or how many studies we consult, we get a different answer. As we have discussed, there are so many different parts of the gut to focus on and surfaces to sample that every analysis gives us a different answer.

However, if we focus on stool samples (as the great majority of studies are on stools), a predominance of bacteria known as *Bacteroides* is typically observed. These species make up a significant proportion of all bacteria found in human stool, accounting for about 25–30 percent. *Bacteroides* are a large group of about fifty closely related species, all of which are anaerobic, non-sporing, and rod-shaped, particularly known for digesting plant carbohydrates.

The familiar *Bifidobacterium* spp. account for another significant proportion of bacteria in the stool, about 10%, and thereafter there is a list

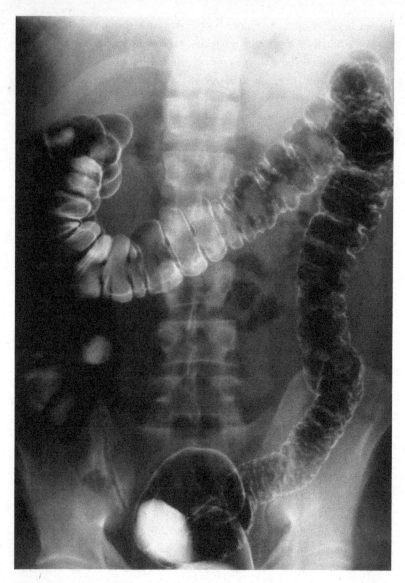

Figure 5.1 Double contrast barium enema X-ray depicting the large intestine (colon) the main site of the gastrointestinal microbiome. Structures visualised include the ascending colon (dimly seen on the left of the image), transverse colon, splenic flexure (top right of the image), descending colon, sigmoid colon and rectum (bottom of the image). Note the mucosal lining of the descending colon has a fine irregular granular mucosal surface due to an infection with *Schistosoma mansoni*.

Source: Wellcome Collection.

including *Lactobacillus* spp. (2 percent), *Clostridium* spp. (2 percent), *Streptococcus* spp. (0.2 percent), Enterobacteriaceae (0.4 percent), and many others in smaller numbers. In all, about 600 bacterial species have been identified in the gut using culture-based techniques.[3,4]

The Enterobacteriaceae, the last group on the list, appears at first glance to be just a loose term for intestinal bacteria (enteric). However, "Enterobacteriaceae" is a formal term denoting a particular family of bacteria. This family includes many important species, some of which are quite familiar, such as *E. coli, klebsiella, shigella,* and *salmonella.* Although as a group they can be said to have certain shared characteristics, such as being rod-shaped, gram-negative, and facultative anaerobes, the term illustrates the difficulty of understanding which bacteria are being referred to at any one time. The Enterobacteriaceae family includes over thirty genera and more than a hundred species, with some being important pathogens and others obscure commensals. But grouping them together and saying that they account for 0.4 percent of the bacteria in a stool sample clearly obscures important details.

Even more baffling is when the analysis is expressed in phyla, which is two levels of organization above families (the rest being domain, kingdom, phylum, class, order, family, genera, and species). At present, there are said to be eight different phyla represented in our stools, with the two main ones being Firmicutes, which apparently make up 50 percent of our gut microbes, and Bacteroidetes, which account for 35 percent. Although at first glance this also seems like a useful way of summarizing a busy data set, just like families (but worse), it is too simplistic. It is a bit like being told that your home or garden has too many vertebrates and not enough arthropods. We might for example, be very happy to be accommodating a rare species of shrew and some Red Admiral butterflies, but maybe not a colony of brown rats or a wasp's nest. Knowing the species makes all the difference, and the theory that too many Bacteroidetes and not enough Firmicutes might be associated with obesity, while popular for a time, is perhaps too sweeping to make sense and is no longer well supported.[5]

The number of bacterial species in the human gut has turned out to be large, even larger than was initially thought from the culture methods.

94 THE MICROBIOME

If we look now at genetic-based research using 16S rRNA analysis, this has expanded our repertoire of gut microbes from 600 to over a thousand. An early study from 2005 illustrating this sudden expansion focused on just three individuals. It identified 395 bacterial species, 244 of which were completely new to science, with the great majority (70 percent) never before cultured. As well as this wealth of new bacteria, a new species of archaea, *Methanobrevibacter smithii*, was also found.[6]

Metagenomic analysis has since expanded the number of bacteria potentially found in the human gut even further, to more than 15,000 species (see note 3). A single paper in 2010 identified 1,150 species in a cohort of just 124. This study found an average of 160 species in each person. As well as identifying more bacteria, metagenomics has also, of course, allowed our focus to widen and include other microbes.[7] A re-analysis of publicly available catalogs of metagenome-assembled genomes claimed to have identified sequences representing fifteen new species of archaea in the human gut.[8]

As well as archaea, the human gut has been found to contain human, animal, and plant viruses, as well as bacteriophages and archaeal viruses, all present in very large numbers—up to a trillion per gram of stool.[9,10]

There are around 267 different fungi that can be present in someone's gut. Examples such as *Candida* spp., *Saccharomyces*, and *Cladosporium* are common. However, there are usually fewer than ten types of fungi in any one person at a time. Their presence is typically very transient, reflecting their probable ingestion on food rather than being a true part of the microbiome. And unlike the skin, the gut also contains protozoa; the commonest one, *Blastocystis* spp., is found in 50 percent of us; others include *Hexamitidae, Trichomonadidae*, and *Entamoeba*. Although these protozoa don't seem to cause disease, even in people with weaker immune systems, they are probably best seen as parasitic.

How Reliable Is Microbiome Research?

Microbiome research on the gut, similar to that on the skin, can be difficult to make sense of, contradictory, and elusive. Even keeping up with the different names, families, and genera of bacteria can be challenging, especially as these names are frequently altered and might have been up-dated anytime from the last century to the last three or four days. In addition to this, many bacteria don't even have proper names yet; the number of new species that metagenomics analysis has uncovered is prodigiously large, and the standard bacterial naming systems are struggling to keep up.

In fact, there is a debate in science as to whether to keep the present system, whereby each bacterium has to be cultured, described, published, and have a type strain kept in a freezer to be distributed to any scientist who wishes to check it, or whether to allow new species to be registered known only from metagenomic sequencing data.

This debate is unresolved, and at present there are two conflicting species registration options acting in parallel. One is willing to accept genetic code, the SeqCode registry (although there is also a healthy debate going on as to what denotes a species based on percentage differences in genetic code—good luck with that one). The other, the International Code of Nomenclature of Prokaryotes (ICNP), accepts cultured species only. Just to add spice to the debate, SeqCode accepts that ICNP is valid too, but ICNP rejects the validity of SeqCode. SeqCode has plenty of support, as scientists are desperate to get some clarity over which bacteria is which. But without actual bacteria to work with, it is hard to take any analysis further.[11]

Apart from not leaving us with an actual bacterium to analyze, metagenomic techniques have other limitations, as we know. The technique cannot reliably identify how many microbes are in a sample, nor whether the bacteria in the sample were originally alive, injured, or dead. It also has no "depth analysis," by which we mean it will miss less-prevalent bacteria completely. These less-prevalent bacteria often include pathogens, but we know they are there and being missed because we can identify them using traditional medical laboratory techniques.

Most seriously though, and not fully acknowledged by the microbiome community, metagenomics has a serious error rate. Depending on the different lab protocols, sequencers, and reagents used, different labs end up with radically different results, which can cause "considerable problems

96 THE MICROBIOME

in the reproducibility of studies and can lead to contradicting results from conceptually similar studies."[12]

Because of this known variability, two specially developed samples have been developed by the World Health Organization (WHO) and the National Institute of Biological Standards and Control (NIBSC) to help standardize results. One sample is of whole bacterial cells, and the other has the DNA already extracted, each containing an exactly known amount of twenty carefully chosen stool bacteria.

Testing these known samples on commercially developed kits has already proved the inherent variation routinely seen with metagenomic techniques. Different results are found for each standard, whether it be DNA per nanogram, specificity, or sensitivity. Some kits pick up 95 percent of the bacteria, while others identify only 20 percent. Some name all of the species correctly, while others only get 70 percent right. Each stage of the analysis appears to add bias, from the DNA extraction (which typically adds a 12-percent error) to the sequence analysis (which adds another 22 percent). If we then add in a sampling bias and a storage bias, it can add up to almost 50 percent of the data being inaccurate.

Following the initial kit testing, these standard samples have been sent out to twenty-two different labs around the world. Early results of this real-world analysis reveal an error rate ranging from 14 to 66 percent. Many labs were not even able to identify a typical gut species, *Ruminococcus* spp., within the sample. Of course, it is natural to have error rates in science; the thing is to acknowledge the error rate and then attempt to correct for it, using carefully developed standards like these. These standard samples are designed to be easily affordable, as WHO wants them to be readily available to any lab that requests them.[13]

The variable nature of metagenomic data and the limitations of not having actual bacteria to work with have been recognized from the beginning. To address this, and starting once again in oceanic science—which, as we have seen, has consistently been at the forefront of these developments— the technique of culturing bacteria has had a complete renaissance. Many previously "unculturable bacteria" have now been cultured. This rejuvenated technique has become known as "culturomics." Taking the lead from oceanic science, which simply used extracts of seawater as a versatile culture medium for bacteria found in the ocean, human researchers have found that different extractions of stool grow all sorts of bacteria really well. Other culture mediums have since been developed, the best of which is an anaerobic mixture of blood mixed with rumen fluid (fluid from the stomach of a ruminant animal).[14]

Hand in hand with the development of culturomics (and it wouldn't have been possible without it) is the Matrix-Assisted Laser Desorption Ionization Time-Of-Flight (MALDI-TOF) mass spectrometer. This amazing piece of equipment has totally streamlined bacterial identification. Instead of a battery of tests to check appearance, staining, preferred growing conditions, biochemistry, and so on for each bacterium, the MALDI-TOF technician simply picks up a small amount of the bacteria colony growing on an agar plate using the pointed tip of a cocktail stick, deposits it on the sample plate in the machine, and presses the On button.

The sample, mixed with a special matrix, is ionized, allowing the proteins in the sample to be separated and the time of flight of each measured (which varies depending on their size). The resulting measurement makes up a sort of protein fingerprint for each species of bacteria, allowing its identification by comparing it to a library of bacteria protein fingerprints. As the machine's library builds up it can identify more and more bacteria with better and better accuracy. Since 2009, MALDI-TOF has revolutionized not just microbiome research but also medical microbiology, enabling five to ten cultured samples to be identified within two to three minutes, compared to hours of testing previously.[15]

Since culturomics has been established, it has not taken long for a head-to-head study to be published comparing culturomics with metagenomics. A study based on three individuals and an epic 212 different culture conditions yielded 340 cultured species. Metagenomic analysis of the same samples revealed just 282 species. Interestingly, only fifty-one overlapped, highlighting gaps in both techniques and clearly showing how tentative any conclusions drawn from either technique has to be.[16]

Traditional microscopy and culture, 16S rRNA analysis, metagenomics, and culturomics are all exciting techniques, each with its own limitations, but each pointing to the vast variety of microbes inside us. Together, these techniques act like a super-strength microscope, allowing us to visualize in detail many of the microbes inside us, although, of course, missing many others.

Although we can see the limitations of each technique, we cannot deny the existence of that huge variety. But now that we know all about the large number of microbes that can potentially be found inside us, we have to start to consider what it all means. We can't continually be satisfied simply by these long lists. We want to know what these lists imply. Where have these microbes come from? What do they do? And is the presence of each meaningful, or are they just on their travels, dividing as they go and having a sort of gap year inside us?

To fully understand the impact microbes are having on each host—whether it is us, mice, rats, flying creatures such as bats, or even insects—the research has to focus on more about each creature than just its microbes. Because although microbes are found inside every animal, we already know that not every animal has the same microbiome. We need to know a creature's intestinal anatomy, its gut transit times, its environmental habitat, and its nutrition before we can make sense of the presence of any microbes we have found. With this kind of information, we can then better determine whether an animal is likely to host and need a microbiome or whether, in fact, it might not have a microbiome, and it has been established some animals don't. The fact that not every animal needs one surely casts some doubts on the claims made for the importance of microbiomes.[17]

How Do We Get the Microbes in Our Gut?

Fortunately, when it comes to humans, we already know our gut anatomy and transit times, where we live, and what we eat, and therefore we have a good idea of where and how we get the microbes in our gut and whether we are hosting a microbiome. Like all creatures we get the microbes in our gut by the simple expedient of swallowing them.

In a way, our gut microbiome is an open ecosystem. The outside world and the world inside us really act as a sort of continuum.[18] We can see this more clearly if we think of a simple organism such as an earthworm. If we visualize the soil surrounding it and then going right through it, we can easily see that continuation of inside and outside. We, too, constantly have microbes from our environment going into our gut and then coming out again and rejoining the outside world. Whenever we breathe and swallow, whatever we eat, and even when we just touch things with our mouths—like our fingers, cups and plates, knives and forks—the microbes attached to those things will get inside of us. When we consider all the microbes we are constantly coming into contact within our environment, it's not surprising that the microbes in our gut are incredibly varied, incredibly numerous and constantly changing. They reflect the vast variety of microbes that surround us.

Just like the earthworm consuming the nutritious particles it finds in the soil, the main thing going through us is our food. Of course, we have to be careful to eat uncontaminated food to avoid food poisoning and food-based infections; this is a constant preoccupation of humans—to avoid food that has gone bad. Our food always has to be fresh or washed or cooked in some way, or preserved by drying, smoking, canning, or fermenting to prevent any mold and spoilage from pathogenic microbes that might cause us to get ill.

But as well as the rare presence of pathogenic bacteria, there are plenty of perfectly benign microbes on our food. Even fresh, unspoiled food has millions of bacteria covering it all over. Most research on food-based microbes is naturally focused on pathogens, but here our interest is just on ordinary bacteria. Analysis of different types of non-pathogenic bacteria found on different foods show a huge variety and every different type of product harbors its own typical set.

Certain foods can be grouped. For example, tree fruits have their own varieties compared to fruits such as strawberries that have had contact with the soil. The microbes on meat are different from the microbes on bread or pasta. Foods such as salami or cheese tend to contain the lactic acid bacteria used in their preservation. Every analysis reveals yet more bacteria, an endless variety on every individual food type.[19]

100 THE MICROBIOME

As well as the varieties of microbes on our food, we can also consider the *number* of microbes found on our food and calculate how many we might consume in one day. Lang et al. analyzed the microbes consumed by a person eating what his team called an average American diet (consisting mainly of convenience foods) and compared it to a US Department of Agriculture–recommended diet (with more fruit and vegetables and leaner meat) and, as well, a vegan diet. Different meals for each diet type were assembled by a dietitian for breakfast, lunch, and dinner, aiming for a total of 2,200 calories per day and cooked in an ordinary kitchen. These meals were then blended, and a 4-milliliter sample was sent to the laboratory for analysis. It was found that a typical American consumes about 1 million to 1 trillion *living* bacteria per day, even more if they eat uncooked or fermented foods.[20]

Although initially alive, these bacteria, once swallowed, as we know, have to endure the hostile environment of the human gut, starting with the intense acidity of the stomach. Many bacteria will be killed outright, and others are damaged or die on their journey. How many of the bacteria that we eat even survive to reach the colon?

Studies where subjects were deliberately given a dose of 100 million *Lactobacillus* bacteria (a lot more of just one bacterium than would ever naturally be consumed in a yogurt drink) found that less than 50 percent survived. Those that did were only present in the stool for a few days and rarely longer than a week.[21]

Other studies that looked for food bacteria that survived the transit, also found some that remained viable, including *Lactococcus lactis, Pediococcus acidilactici*, and *Streptococcus thermophilus*—all bacteria frequently found on the surface of meats and cheeses. Additionally, fungi such as *Candida, Debaryomyces, Penicillium*, and *Scopulariopsis*, which commonly colonize vegetables, were found, and even a plant virus (a spinach pathogen).[22]

The endlessly variable nature of our gut microbes seems to perfectly reflect the transient and endlessly variable microbes that are found on our foods.

Are There Microbes in Our Tap Water?

We absolutely depend on our tap water for safe drinking water and hygiene purposes and might therefore assume it is perfectly clean; after all it's there for washing with. But although our tap water may look clear and taste fine, it is not, in fact, free from microbes. As well as eating a trillion microbes a day on our food, it appears that we also unknowingly drink them.

Just as with eating, where we are able to tolerate consuming a certain number of microbes on the food, we are also able to tolerate a certain number of microbes in our drinking water. The predominant species in tap water—*Acinetobacter* spp., *Aeromonas* spp., *Alcaligenes* spp., *Comamonas* spp., *Enterobacter* spp., *Flavobacterium* spp., *Klebsiella* spp., *Moraxella* spp., *Pseudomonas* spp., *Sphingomonas* spp., and *Stenotrophomonas* spp. (here listed alphabetically like a fiendishly difficult children's rhyme)—are not usually individually identified when checking water samples. Rather the whole lot is cultured for forty-eight hours at a temperature of 20 degrees centigrade (with the exact times, temperatures, and agar gels varying according to the latest guidelines), and the rate of colony-forming units (CFU) per milliliter is counted. Every bacterium is counted, no matter which sort. This nonspecific water count is known as a heterotrophic plate count, with "heterotrophic" referring to the varied collection of bacteria living off organic material suspended in the water.

In America, as well as in many European countries (and alongside other water safety tests), water with less than 100 CFU per milliliter is considered very pure, 100−500 open to suspicion, and over 1,000 implies that the water source is probably contaminated, usually by sewage. These ranges were established right at the start of bacteriology by Koch in 1892. At this time, the Elbe River near Hamburg had become contaminated with cholera bacteria, leading to a cholera outbreak in Hamburg and the deaths of 7,000 people. However, Koch established that those living in nearby Altona, who used the same contaminated water but filtered, were fine. He proposed the limit of 100 CFU per milliliter as safe and famously said that "when all was said and done, he, personally, would rather not drink this filtered water at all. Yet one had to live with uncertainty, to trust something less than rigorous demonstration, and be satisfied with estimates of risk."

If we drink, on average, 2 liters of tap water every twenty-four hours, we can calculate that each day we probably drink about 200,000 microbes of every sort, including pathogens. Bottled water, in contrast reaches levels of 100,000 CFU per milliliter once bottled, as disinfection or chemical treatment of natural mineral water is not permitted, meaning those aficionados of bottled water are drinking more microbes, not less, than if they stick to tap water.[23] But it may be reassuring to know that although we are drinking pathogens every day, we would need to swallow a pretty large dose of any disease-causing microbes to get an infection. For instance, we would need to ingest 10,000 *Mycobacterium avium* to make us truly ill, and in the case of *Pseudomonas aeruginosa* microbes, a trillion.[24]

Do We Get Gut Microbes from our Toilets?

Toilets are yet another source of microbes and perhaps one more to the point with regard to our colon microbiomes. Although toilets significantly reduce rates of fecal-oral disease by effectively separating us from our stools, they are not perfectly efficient at this task.

To test the spread of bacteria from toilets, a liquid formulation of a benign bacterium was formulated to simulate diarrheal illness. A sample with a known number of bacteria was squirted into each toilet basin and the toilet flushed. It was found that the flush neatly dispersed the bacteria into the air, and that then after a certain amount of time, the bacteria settled on various bathroom surfaces—the sink, the floor near the toilet, and especially the toilet seat. Closing the toilet lid made no difference. The gap between the lid and the seat that prevents us from pinching our fingers allows a jet of air to project the bacteria straight into the bathroom, just as efficiently as when the lid is up.

Reassuringly though, the flush does make a difference to the bacteria in the toilet water. Every flush reduces the number of bacteria by a thousandfold, rapidly reducing the level of viable bacteria to less than 1,000 CFU milliliter and reducing the potential spread of diarrheal disease.[25]

On the one hand, knowing about stool bacteria being dispersed into the air by our toilets may make us think a bit more about brushing our teeth, especially if our toothbrush has been lying around in the kind of modern bathroom that combines a toilet with a sink and a bath. On the other hand, if we see these microbes as useful to our health, then in a way our bathrooms may be helpful in facilitating their transfer. Microbes that find it hard to survive, such as anaerobic bacteria, may be more likely to make it to the next person if they have been conveniently catapulted out of a toilet and straight onto someone's face sponge or flannel. If the microbe survives this transit and its journey through the bowel, it could potentially become the next long-term inhabitant of our colons.

Do the Nutrients in Our Diet Affect Our Microbiomes?

As we have seen, different varieties of bacteria are constantly entering our gastrointestinal system on the food that we eat, the water that we drink, and the things that come into contact with our mouths. But it's also important to be clear that microbial gut populations also rise and fall with the nutrients in the foods that we eat. Each food provides a nutrient perfect for a certain bacteria to thrive, potentially leading to a boom in their population.

As we saw with the neonatal microbiome, where there was milk, there would be a bloom of *Bifidobacterium*, but the same is true of any nutrient. If we eat more meat, we find all of a sudden that we have more *Acinetobacter* and *Clostridium*; more vegetables, we find more *Bacteroides* and *Prevotella*; and with more sugar, more *Enterococcus*. There is a large range of different bacteria that can digest each nutrient, and this goes another long way to explain the massive variety of bacterial species seen within each of our gut microbiomes.

How Can We Make Sense of the Gut Microbiome If the Microbes in It Are So Variable?

But what are we to conclude from all of this? Although we now have an extensive list of known gut microbes and an understanding of how we get these gut microbes, we still don't have a sense of how important any one

104 THE MICROBIOME

microbe is, if indeed any are. The Human Microbiome Project was going to describe the gut microbiome in particular once and for all and work out what a "normal microbiome" was. From there, it would have been a short step to start considering therapeutic uses. But it hasn't worked out like that. The main discovery of the Human Microbiome Project is how variable each person's microbiome is, whether from the nose, mouth, skin, gut, or urogenital tract. No normal gut microbiome has been identified, just this immense variety. We are still very much in the dark.

To try to pin down the meaning of this variability, very large trials are being generated. As well as collecting stool samples and noting down basic parameters such as age and sex, as the initial studies did, these trials are making extensive efforts to get a much more detailed idea of each person's personal or observable characteristics, their lifestyle and their environment. From this it may be possible to work out if any of these factors are associated with a particular microbe.

A good example of this kind of trial is the Dutch Microbiome Project. This includes over 8,000 individuals in various households, some with up to three generations. This study has documented all sorts of parameters: pet ownership, whether the person is retired, their alcohol intake, whether they live in a green space or urban, the local nitrogen dioxide concentration, pregnancy, smoking history, fat intake, protein intake, and so on, as well as taking multiple samples from each person.

But although a massive 241 parameters have been analyzed, these have only explained around 15 percent of the interindividual variation in microbiome composition, a result fairly consistent with other large studies. This leaves 85 percent of the variation as unexplained or possibly simply irrelevant, either representing transient microbes or other microbes not having an obvious impact. This kind of fits with the idea that the gut is open to all comers and that a lot of the species picked up are simply passing through or indeed already dead.[26]

Even so, the hunt is still on to try to find an association between gut microbiome profiles and something useful. As well as looking at these multiple parameters, many studies have focused on a particular disease and its association with the gut microbiome. Apparent differences in gut microbiomes are frequently picked up in different disease states, especially gastrointestinal diseases such as ulcerative colitis, Crohn's disease, and irritable bowel syndrome, or even conditions that are not primarily gastrointestinal, such as rheumatoid arthritis and multiple sclerosis. It is usual, at the very least, to notice a decrease in bowel microbe diversity associated with reduced health in each condition. So far, though, it has not been established in any case whether a disease has caused an altered microbiome (the most likely scenario) or whether an altered microbiome has caused the disease.

To answer this chicken-and-egg conundrum, even larger, more expensive longitudinal studies are being undertaken around the world. The American Gut Project and the UK Biobank are just two examples; the multinational Human Phenotype Project is another, aiming to collect phenotypic data from a massive 100,000 individuals (although its early days, and they have so far reached approximately 9,000). This data will then be linked with both microbiome data and an extensive range of ordinary medical tests. The very long timeframe means that as the years pass some subjects will inevitably develop diabetes, cancer, or some other medical disease, and it will then be possible to track any change to the microbiome as it happens, answering once and for all whether a change to the microbiome causes a disease or the other way round.

Is There a Core Microbiome?

A core microbiome is a set of key microbes that all of us would have inside us. Whether there is a core microbiome is the hundred-million-dollar question and the holy grail of microbiome research. If we only knew which the key gut microbes were, we could manufacture them and then truthfully sell them as being essential to human health.

Multiple efforts are constantly being made to identify a core microbiome; in one study nine species were identified as being present in more than 95 percent of individuals: *Subdoligranulum sp.*, *Alistipes onderdonkii*, *Alistipes putredinis*, *Alistipes shahii*, *Bacteroides uniformis*, *Bacteroides vulgatus*, *Eubacterium rectale*, *Faecalibacterium prausnitzii*, and *Oscillibacter sp.* This result is highly consistent with other studies done in the United Kingdom, the United States, and Europe (see note 26). Another study, GutFeelingKB, has developed a different list that includes 109 species.[27] Yet another study, the Gut Microbiome Health Index, is based on fifty species and is now being developed as a test to identify "non-healthy" stools. These studies assume that we are all talking about the same thing when we use the term "core microbiome." But are we?

The studies quoted above seem to assume that the core microbiome should include the microbes most commonly found within a host population. This is sometimes known as the "common core." A common core is usually defined as including the microbes that occur above a particular occupancy frequency threshold, usually asserted to be anywhere between 30 percent and 95 percent, although there is no particular biological justification for such a threshold. Theoretically, a core microbe like this would have to be present in quite high numbers, but it may still have no specific effect on our health. It could simply be common because it is prevalent in the environment, prevalent in the host's diet, or simply because that microbe outcompetes others in the gut.

A different kind of core microbe could be one that is stable over time: a "temporal core." This sort might still be there after a year or even five years later, or it might be there at certain times of the year or at certain stages of the host's life cycle. It could either be rare or found in large numbers. However, a temporal core microbe could be consistently present simply because of the "priority effect"—it got there first. This would lead to a microbiome that is highly stable and resistant to invasion by other microbes, but still might have absolutely no effect on the host.

If at this stage we consider a microbial example, say *Bacteroides* spp., which account for 20–30 percent of microbes in human stool, we could consider this microbe as being in both a common and a temporal core. We know this species digests carbohydrates. We might then wonder if this bacteria could be having an effect on our health? A microbe that genuinely had an effect on host function would be described as being in a "functional core."

But a really exciting core microbe would be one that both affected our health (like the functional core) but also had a function that simply couldn't be done by any other microbe: the "host-adapted core."

These would be the microbes that we might have co-evolved with. They would probably have to be vertically transmitted (mother to baby) and be present in large numbers to ensure reliable transmission.[28] *Bifidobacteria* spp., the microbe that we found was so prevalent in neonates across the world, could be a contender for this kind of co-evolved bacteria. However, as we know, some babies do not have it at all and appear to be fine. However we define it—whether common, temporal, functional, or host-adapted—identifying a core gut microbiome in adult humans has so far proven elusive.

Does Our Gut Microbiome Affect Our Calorie Intake?

Even if we can't identify the exact microbes that make up a core microbiome (if one even exists in humans), we can still consider what the microbes inside our colon are doing: whether they are simply consuming nutrients and living inside us as parasites or, the opposite, processing our hard-to-digest food remnants and helping us to extract more calories from our diet.

It is known from people who have had surgery to remove their small intestine that, although the colon mainly absorbs fluids and salts, it can, if needed, absorb short- and medium-chain fatty acids. Many bacteria are known to produce short-chain fatty acids (SCFAs). Do the bacteria in the colon produce enough SCFAs to make a significant difference to our energy intake?

This is a hard question to answer, and there is no evidence in humans that we can draw upon, except anatomical; we have a colon that allows bacteria to multiply, which must give us some evolutionary advantage, otherwise it would not be there.

Experiments in rats do show a possible effect on calorie intake. Where conventional rats appear to extract 80 percent of the nutrients from their food, germ-free rats extract only 71.9 percent.[29] However, the energy required to both contain and yet keep up a barrier between us and our gut microbes takes its toll too and evens up the energy equation. Groups of germ-free rats in the same weight range as groups of conventional rats are found to need the same or, if anything, less food overall on a daily basis, even though they can perhaps extract slightly fewer calories from their food.[30]

108 THE MICROBIOME

But let's suppose that we are similar to rats (both of us being omnivores, although we don't eat our poop and extract further nutrients from it as they do) and assume that microbes allow us to extract an additional 8 percent of calories from our food, as rats seem to.

At first glance, that does not seem like a big deal. We can easily eat an extra four-finger KitKat a day and immediately get more than an additional 8 percent of our calories in just a few mouthfuls. In today's calorie-rich world, 160 calories is neither here nor there (in fact, the challenge is usually to avoid accidentally eating an additional 160 calories). There is no doubt that as individuals and from a calorie point of view most of us simply don't need a microbiome right now for extracting extra energy.

But imagine we were living in a less food-rich environment. In medieval England in the early 11th century, famines are recorded as occurring on average every four years, and people at this time were obsessed with preserving food. To have a repository of food was not just wealth, it was essential to survival. If we lived at this time, an extra 8 percent of calories would be a boon. During a difficult year, an extra 8 percent of calories still might not have been enough for some very poor peasants to survive, and others, more well off, wouldn't have needed it. But to that exact group of people just on the edge of starvation, it would have been just enough to help them make it through and survive to die another day. For a population, to have a colon with bacteria working away giving extra calories would be a genuine survival advantage, an evolutionary pressure.[31]

The variation in gut microbes found between humans appears to suggest that we have evolved a "functional core" microbiome, one that allows us to absorb extra calories but one in which it appears that any plant, carbohydrate, or meat-digesting microbes will do.

Do All Animals Have a Microbiome?

In contrast to most mammals that have evolved to co-opt microbes, some animals have evolved to simply tolerate microbes. Certain types of omnivorous ants, but also caterpillars, butterflies, and dragonflies, do not have a microbiome at all. Of course, they have microbes in them, but these are just passing through, attached to whatever they have eaten that day, and are in no way necessary to the creature's survival.[32]

Other animals vary in their dependence on microbes to affect calorie intake. Whereas carnivores or omnivores like us have no difficulty extracting the great majority of calories and nutrients we need from our food directly from the stomach and small intestine without much help from a microbiome, plant eaters cannot.

Herbivores such as guinea pigs and rabbits, which are hindgut fermenters, absorb most of their food in the stomach and gut, extracting just a little bit extra by fermenting the semi-digested food in the cecum, passing it as pellets, and then eating it. Not having a microbiome affects their food absorption a bit.

In contrast, ruminant animals such as goats and cows are foregut fermenters. They have not one stomach but four; the first three are for fermenting the food with bacteria, while the last is for absorbing nutrients. Not having a microbiome would presumably affect them a lot but it hasn't been possible to raise a ruminant animal in germ-free conditions for longer than a few weeks.

Can Germ-Free Animals Absorb Their Food Properly?

Research on germ-free animals has been going on for over a century now, but it is well recognized that initially the specialty was beset by problems to do with nutrition. The ways of sterilizing food available in the 1900s, such as steaming or boiling, destroyed many essential nutrients, most of which were not even known about at this time. Consequently, germ-free animals initially suffered from various nutrient deficiencies. The revelations about micronutrients and vitamins achieved during the first part of the 20th century and later revolutions in sterilizing food by using radiation and filtration instead of the earlier methods, finally allowed germ-free animals to live a healthy life, and scientists could then study germ-free animals properly, over their full life span.

110 THE MICROBIOME

We already know that germ-free animals look alright from the outside, live longer than conventional animals and can even reproduce effectively. But although fascinating, this is not quite enough to satisfy us. Extensive research has been done on germ-free animals to further understand how they function without a microbiome.

The simple answer is that although germ free animals can absorb their food properly, they are a little bit different. They necessarily have to be. As a creature that has evolved to cope with microbes, whether the effect of microbes is mainly detrimental or mainly beneficial or a bit of both, removing all the microbes is bound to have an effect. It can cause some problems and, conversely, it can lead to some nutritional advantages.[33]

It turns out that since the microbes are not there, they don't digest the bile and pancreatic enzymes produced by the body in their usual way; so, nutrient absorption in germ-free animals is actually significantly more efficient. If given a calorie-restricted diet, germ-free animals are more likely to maintain a healthy weight. In addition, germ-free animals have more efficient calcium and magnesium absorption, leading to measurably heavier and stronger bones. They also absorb certain essential amino acids more effectively than conventional animals, which we will revisit in the gut-brain chapter.

If we consider the absorption of micronutrients such as vitamin K or vitamin C, we can see that the effect of the microbiome is not necessarily beneficial and can indeed be detrimental. Vitamin K is an essential vitamin that helps us with blood clotting. Although many sources assure us that a gut microbiome is essential for our vitamin K production, in actual fact the contribution of microbes to our vitamin K levels is very slight. Most of our vitamin K is obtained from dietary fats. In fact, it's not even certain that the microbial form of this product is bioactively available at the cellular level.

If we compare germ-free rats to conventional rats maintained on a vitamin K-free diet, they show a tendency to bleed and succumb to vitamin K deficiency illness only about a week before a conventional rat, showing a real—but very marginal—disadvantage. It is likely that microbes, which also require vitamin K to survive, are simply producing it for their own needs.[34]

In contrast, if we consider vitamin C, we know that microbes also need this vitamin and, like us, have to obtain it from dietary sources—in other words, from us, their host, from our diet. Although a germ-free animal on a very low vitamin C diet will live a healthy life indefinitely, a conventional animal on the same diet will die of vitamin C deficiency and scurvy within two weeks, implying that the gut microbiome is scavenging vitamin C from the intestinal contents to the detriment of the host.

Can We Lose Microbes from Our Gut Microbiome?

Can we lose variety in our gut microbiome? Say we entirely cut out carbohydrates, would we lose the carbohydrate-digesting bacteria? And if we did, does it matter? The answer is yes; if we cut out certain foods, such as carbohydrates, there will be a temporary reduction in carbohydrate-digesting bacteria. But when we eat carbohydrates again, they will effortlessly bloom and recover.

But if over time we really didn't eat any carbohydrates, not one bit, would the carbohydrate-consuming bacteria go completely? The answer is yes; we would lose some bacterial species permanently. Mice fed a low microbiota-accessible-carbohydrate (MAC) diet that doesn't support the populations of certain bacteria, really do gradually lose species and end up with a simplified gut microbiome. In one study, 141 out of 208 bacteria in these animals vanished completely within four generations, and reintroduction of the lost nutrients was insufficient to regain those lost bacteria.[35]

Of course, if this had happened to us, perhaps through dietary alterations, antiseptic cleaning products, or overuse of antibiotics—we know that we would be able to get these bacteria back again from our environment and from other people. But if these bacteria did not remain in the vicinity, just like those mice, we would not be able to get them back and could potentially lose them forever.

We can see this loss happen in real life to children suffering from malnutrition. In these children, who have not had access to adequate nutrients, the stool bacteria are found to be rather simplified. The usual variety of

112 THE MICROBIOME

hundreds of species is measurably reduced, as if they were younger than they actually are and haven't yet accumulated a full set of microbes. Even when these children are re-fed with nutritious foods, they do not thrive or gain weight as quickly as they should, and their stools remain depleted of the usual variety of microbes.[36]

The lack of a normal diverse stool microbiome in malnourished children and its apparent impact on growth when these children are re-fed is one of the first proven instances of the microbiome having a real impact and a real medical use. To potentially aid in the weight gain of malnourished children is a really significant therapeutic use of our knowledge of the microbiome. It's a genuinely exciting moment.

Ongoing studies are still being designed in Bangladesh to combine refeeding with microbe supplements, either by considering the microbes on the foods selected for refeeding or as an additional live biotherapeutic supplement. A certain refeeding formulation that includes chickpea flour, soy flour, peanut flour, and banana flour shows distinct advantages over the standard Ready to Use Supplementary Food (RUSF).[37]

Does Our Fiber Intake Affect Our Gut Microbes?

The foods we eat clearly have a major impact on our microbiome, both from the bacteria on the food and for the bacteria already in the gut scavenging the food. As we have seen, adding nutrients to the diet can lead to big blooms of microbes in the gut, and removal of nutrients to some microbes dying out altogether.

However, some species are more robust. These are microbes that typically digest fiber. They have a cunning survival mechanism, a secret weapon: an alternative food source. If given a fiber-free diet (not uncommon in our industrial world), these bacteria simply turn to digesting intestinal mucus.

We have already encountered intestinal mucus and seen its protective effect as the lining of the gut in our journey through the intestinal tract. Our mucus acts to separate the gut microbes from the epithelial cells lining our intestines in the same way as the layers of dead corneocytes separate the microbes in the environment from our skin cells. There are scientists who have spent their entire lives analyzing the amazing qualities of intestinal mucus, building on earlier research from the 1970s by scientists who spent *their* entire lives on it. They have studied its chemical make-up, its antimicrobial properties, its hourly turnover, and the anatomy of its inner and outer layers.[38] Our intestinal mucus goes a long way in explaining how our gastrointestinal tract can digest food and yet not digest itself. It also explains how the gastrointestinal tract can safely contain a high load of microbes without overloading the immune system. Acting like a kind of force field, this constantly renewed transparent barrier simply separates the microbes from the epithelial cells, avoiding unnecessary inflammation.

Stains of the inner layer of mucus show that the mucosal cell surface is typically bacteria-free. Of course, the odd bacterium does get through to this surface, but it is usually quickly dispatched by the immune system. The only time that this area is invaded is when intestinal pathogens with extra abilities to drill through the mucus or consume it in some way, bypass the barrier and cause a gastrointestinal infection.

Although the inner mucus layer is known to be relatively impervious to bacteria, bacteria can clearly be shown in the outer layer of mucus. It is well known that the looser outer layer serves both as a habitat and partial food source for these specialized bacteria that can digest it, including *Bacteroides thetaiotaomicron* and *Akkermansia muciniphila*. Scanning electron microscopy has even revealed little island communities of bacteria assembled on small particles of shed mucus on their way to being excreted. Although these bacteria prefer to digest dietary fiber where they can, if coping with a fiber-poor diet, they will slowly and laboriously digest the mucus glycans instead.[39]

The integrity of the mucus layer is critical for our health. Studies on flies show that if the mucus barrier degrades, the intestinal bacteria start to attack the epithelial cells, leading to an increased immune response, impaired healing, aging, and death.[40] Genetically altered mice bred to have no mucus at all also have greatly increased rates of intestinal inflammation and colon cancer. Mice given reduced dietary fiber in their diet have a thinner colonic mucus, and it is known that mice given a low-fiber diet have a microbiome that damages the mucus barrier.[41]

114 THE MICROBIOME

Maybe it is not an abnormal gut microbiome that we should be concerned about at all, but an abnormal gastrointestinal mucus barrier. Just as damage to the skin barrier by soap disrupts the body's ability to fend off microbes, leading to skin inflammation, so in the gut it appears that damage to the mucus barrier from microbes that don't have enough dietary fiber to consume disrupts the gut's ability to keep the gut microbiome safely contained and leads to intestinal inflammation.

Although we will come to probiotics and other therapeutic treatments for the microbiome in the probiotic chapter, perhaps therapies such as oral fiber to preserve our mucus barrier should be our goal rather than vainly trying to replenish and preserve our highly variable and already well-populated gut microbiome. If we could just eat enough fiber to keep our mucus digesting microbes occupied, they would be too busy and well fed to destroy our mucus barrier.

There are lots of great reasons to keep fiber in our diet (helps us form soft stools, helps us to control blood sugar levels, helps us in achieving a healthy weight), but we can now add in that it appears it may also help to preserve our gut barrier function and reduce inflammation. It is fiber, not a "balanced gut microbiome," that maybe the real key here, to help us live a longer, healthier life.

6

THE MICROBIOME AND THE BRAIN

One of the most popular aspects of the microbiome is the idea that our gut microbes can affect our minds in some way. In fact, some sources assert that gut microbes control our minds to such an extent that they tell us what foods we should eat, when to exercise or even affect our mental outlook.

Dramatic studies are quoted by the press linking the high prevalence of psychiatric disorders to our gut microbes, depleted due to our modern lifestyles. There are papers that suggest developmental conditions such as autism are linked to the microbes in our diet, and we are advised that the right sort of nutrition will improve it. The gut microbiome has been linked with stress, anxiety, depression, Parkinson's, dementia, alcoholism, ADHD, autism, and nearly every other mental health, aging, addiction, or developmental condition in between.

That a mental health disorder might be due to an imbalance of gut microbes and can be treated with certain foods seems so natural and simple somehow. There is something very attractive about the idea of our gut microbes affecting our mood and being able to cure ourselves with careful attention to what we eat. Linked with modern dietary concepts such as eating whole food, home cooking, and avoiding ultra-processed foods, it all seems to make sense and fit together.

But although the idea is persuasive, or maybe because of this, it may have been oversold. Research papers have tended to give sweeping assertions about the relevance of their findings to mental health issues, journalists have amplified the hyperbole, and the general public have latched on to what seems to be the elegant idea of treating serious mental health or

116 THE MICROBIOME

developmental disorders with careful attention to fiber, fermented foods, probiotics, and fecal transplants.

Extensive claims by scientists describing the power of the microbiome to affect our minds have not helped. "Gut microbiota have developed ways to hack into our reward system to make us crave certain foods and avoid others that are most beneficial to them."[1] "Key findings show that the microbiota is necessary for normal stress responsivity, anxiety-like behaviours, sociability and cognition."[2] "The gut microbiota has emerged as a master regulator of this axis. Thus, opportunities to exploit the microbiome to treat stress-related psychiatric disorders are materializing."[3]

These are big claims. Gut microbes as "master regulators," "hacking" into our reward centers might make us start to wonder if we are still us. Are we just some sort of human puppet controlled by the microbes within us?

So where did it all start? Who first had the idea that gut microbes affect the brain, and how did this morph into concepts of microbes "controlling" our brains? And most importantly, is it true?

The idea of the microbiome affecting the gut-brain axis is often quoted as starting in 2004 with a paper by a scientist named Sudo. Sudo's experiment was conducted on a small group of germ-free mice that were then compared to a small group of specific-pathogen-free (SPF) mice. These mice were deliberately stressed by restraining them, and then their cortisol levels (a stress hormone) were measured and compared.

From this small experiment, a large conclusion was made: that colonizing microbes altered the hypothalamic-pituitary-adrenal (HPA) axis response to stress. The authors asserted that this indicated that the interaction of gut bacteria with the brain was bidirectional. "To our knowledge, this is the first report that shows commensal microbes affecting the neural network responsible for controlling stress responsiveness."

You may be surprised at this point to find out that all of those big claims quoted above about the microbiome affecting the brain are predicated on this small study on mice. When looking at exciting claims made for various microbiome-gut-brain studies, it is always undeniably disappointing to read halfway down and then discover the word "murine," (mouse).

However, in spite of this limitation, Sudo's small study has been hugely influential. Many subsequent studies on gut microbes and mouse behavior have been inspired by this paper, and it has been cited over 2,798 times and counting. For us, trying to understand its sweeping conclusions, and the strange attachment the press has to gut microbes affecting our mental processes, it may have thrown up more questions than it answered.

How Long Have We Known about the Link between the Gut and the Brain?

This may have been the first time that someone asserted that intestinal microbes might affect our "neural network," but it is certainly not the first time anyone has linked the gut and the brain.

We know through experience that simply thinking about food can affect our gut function. That strong and sometimes instant link between our guts and our brains is obvious to all of us. Within seconds of anticipating lunch, we can hear our stomach growling. Similarly, we know that our gut can somehow communicate with our brain, so that we can become suddenly consciously aware that we need food, right now. This is the "bidirectional nature" of the gut-brain axis, the communication runs in both directions and can both activate or dampen down digestion.

There is also a strong emotional link between the gut and the brain. We may have noticed that when we are anxious, we have no appetite, or when we are suddenly frightened, we can get instant diarrhea. Similarly, if we have not eaten, we may feel angry or irritable. Knowledge of the link between our emotions and the gut is longstanding, and it has been documented at least since the 14th century that the "bowels were regarded as the seat of our tender and sympathetic emotions."[4]

By the mid-18th century, physicians were developing theories about how different parts of the body were linked based on extensive anatomical study. The gut especially was noted to have an abundance of nerve endings. Robert Whytt (1714–1766), a Scottish physician, believed that these numerous nerve endings dispensed "nervous energy" throughout the body, and many doctors took on this holistic idea of "nervous sympathy."

118 THE MICROBIOME

During the 19th century, physicians attributed all sorts of mental symptoms to a disordered digestion, such as lowness of spirits, poor sleep, weariness, and fatigue. They recommended simple, natural foods as a remedy.[5] But although at this time doctors blamed the gut for its effect on the mind, as the century progressed the situation reversed. Early 20th-century psychiatrists began to blame the mind for its effect on the gut, noticing the association of anxiety or stress with conditions such as irritable bowel syndrome and stomach ulcers.[6]

It is clear that the link between the gut and the brain (with the added wrinkle of the microbiome), although presented by the microbiome world as new, radical, and offering huge potential for a better understanding of our bodies and our mental health, is neither new nor radical, but in fact well-known, with an extensive scientific basis. It is known today as the gut-brain axis.

What Is the Gut-Brain Axis?

The gut-brain axis is the physical connection between our gut and our brain (see Figure 6.1). These two organs are extensively connected by both nerves, hormones, and metabolically. These connections are multiple, instantaneous, and strong, and, like all systems in the body, have delicate feedback mechanisms so that a signal is started when it is needed and finished when it is not. Once we have seen the gut-brain axis in action, the *microbiome*-gut-brain axis (if it exists at all) must necessarily seem to have a minor role to play.

Our brain and nerves can be thought of in two divisions. The first is our conscious nervous system, where we decide what we are looking at, where we are going, and what food we will eat. The other system is our unconscious nervous system. This one is known as the autonomic system, and it does everything else. It regulates our breathing, our heart pumping, and our intestinal movements.

In fact, the part of the autonomic nervous system involved in the gut is so large that it has its own name: the enteric nervous system. Just as the Scottish physician Robert Whytt noted, it has a huge number of nerve endings,

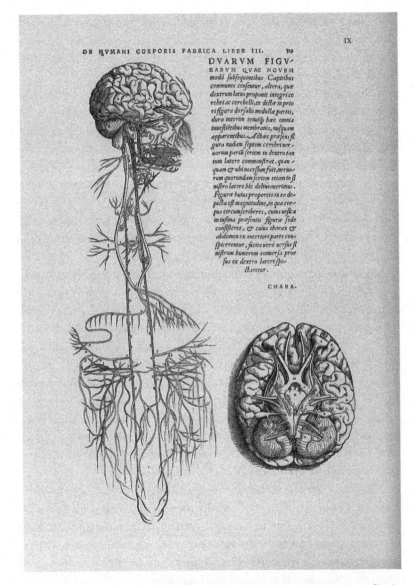

Figure 6.1 Photolithograph, 1940, after a woodcut from 1543 of the brain, in right profile, depicting the major nerves involved in the gut-brain axis, the glossopharyngeal and vagus nerves, and to the right, a view of the base of the brain.

Source: Wellcome Collection.

more than the rest of the body combined. There are sensory and motor nerve endings in every part of the intestinal tract, from mouth to anus and absolutely every inch in between, embedded into the layers of the gut –just under the surface of the epithelial cells.

The enteric system connects with the brain and spine via the prevertebral ganglia nerves (placed just in front of the aorta) for its "fight and flight" signals and via the vagus (a large and important nerve that comes out of the lower part of our brains) for its "rest and digest" signals, a nerve that we will come back to shortly.

Of course, all of these huge numbers of nerve endings need a lot of neurotransmitter chemicals like acetylcholine, dopamine, and serotonin. In fact, the number of nerves in the enteric system is so large that over 95 percent of serotonin, a key neurotransmitter in the body, is found here in the gut (twenty times as much as is found in the brain).

As well as the enormous number of nerves *physically* connecting the gut and the brain, there is also a hormone system *chemically* connecting the two together, in particular the HPA axis, which is part of the endocrine system. This is the endocrine stress axis that Sudo talks about in his paper.

The hypothalamus (the "H" of the HPA axis) is a small organ right in the middle of the brain, and just below it is the pituitary gland (the "P"), another small organ also right in the midline of the brain. Meanwhile the adrenals (the "A" and the final part of the axis) consist of two small organs, each sat on top of a kidney. The hypothalamus makes a hormone that triggers the pituitary, the pituitary makes a hormone that triggers the adrenals, and the adrenals make cortisol, a special hormone particularly linked to stress and the chemical that Sudo measures in his stressed-out mice.

The more stressed we are, the more cortisol we are supposed to make. But as well as getting a surge of cortisol when we are stressed, it's normal to have a surge of cortisol in the morning when we get up as part of our diurnal rhythm, a surge of cortisol when we exercise, and even a surge when we have a viral infection. It is worth noting too that other hormones are produced when we are stressed that Sudo doesn't measure.

Cortisol doesn't appear to act directly on the gut, but it does increase our blood sugar when it is low, and like all endocrine systems, there has to be a break in the system, a way of stopping the cycle. Cortisol does this. It acts on both the hypothalamus and the pituitary and stops them producing their hormones, and this stops the adrenals producing more cortisol.

The nervous system and the endocrine system clearly connect the brain and the gut rapidly and comprehensively, but these two are not the only connections between the gut and the brain. They work closely with the metabolic system, which comes to the forefront once we start eating—or in fact before that, when we start seeing, smelling, or even just thinking about food. As soon as we anticipate a meal, the secretory cells in the stomach are triggered to produce digestive juices. In particular, the enterochromaffin cells secrete histamine, and other cells in the stomach secrete gastrin, acid, and protein-digesting enzymes.

As well as secreting histamine, enterochromaffin cells are also known for secreting serotonin, that important neurotransmitter that we mentioned earlier. Serotonin mediates many functions in the gut, including peristalsis, gastric secretions, vasoconstriction, and the perception of pain and nausea.[7]

As we begin to eat and the food enters our stomachs, the acid and digesting chemicals can get to work on it. Even food coming into actual physical contact with secretory cells can trigger them to make more acid. As the stomach distends in order to hold our meal, the lining stretches, and this sends more signals to the cells in the stomach to make more acid and more gastrin, which make the parietal cells make yet more acid.

This epic acid-producing merry-go-round feedback cycle can't go on forever. Eventually the intense acidity is picked up by chemical sensors, which produce a special hormone to stop all the cells producing acid. Nor can we go on eating forever. The concept of satiety is signaled from the stomach via the vagus nerve to the brain and gives us a conscious feeling of fullness and satisfaction and the impulse to stop eating.

Of course, this is just a sketch of how the initial phases of digestion work, but it's plain to see how instantaneous, interconnected, and finely tuned the gut-brain axis is. From gastric secretions to feedback cycles, we can see how smoothly the metabolic systems interact with the enteric nervous system

122   THE MICROBIOME

and the endocrine system to activate every single part of our gastrointestinal tract into a smooth-running and effective digestion machine.

Do the Gut and the Brain Work Differently in Germ-Free Mice?

Given this intense, powerful, and instant connection of the gut-brain axis, how do the gut microbes fit in? They are there, of course, in the gut, mainly in the colon. And they are affected by every meal, every phase of digestion, and every perturbation of the gastrointestinal system. It is clear that the gut-brain axis has a huge effect on the life of these microbes, but is the directionality both ways? Will the microbes have an effect on the functioning of the gut-brain axis?

We know already that the gut microbes enjoy various activities while in our gut. We know that they ferment plant fibers, releasing certain calories, and that when they don't have enough fiber, they digest our intestinal mucus. We also know that as bacteria, they can activate our immune system. But do they do anything else to affect our physiology? Do they have a direct effect on our brains?

To try to figure this out, it may be interesting at this point to return to our germ-free animals and see what effect there is on the gut-brain axis when animals don't have any microbiome at all.

But although germ-free animals have been studied fully and extensively for many years and with a focus on every single organ—macroscopically, microscopically, and physiologically—did anyone look at the behavior of germ-free animals? Do germ free animals develop normally? Do they interact normally? Because to answer the question, does the microbiome have an effect on the brain, we really want to know what germ-free animals are actually like.

The answer appears to be no, they didn't. Gordon, Coates, and Wostmann—all big writers about germ-free mice who spent decades, if not their whole lives, studying germ-free animals—do not mention behavioral characteristics in germ-free mice, rats, chickens, rabbits, or guinea pigs at any point. There are chapters on the liver, the gut, the immune system, and indeed every system in the body, but not behavior.[8,9,10]

Perhaps the question did not occur to them. The one thing writers on germ-free animals are clear about is that those areas of the body that are protected or walled off from the microbiome—the muscles, the endocrine organs, and, of course, the brain—are the least altered, whereas those organs in close contact with the microbiome, such as the gut and the immune system, are the most affected.

It was not until after Sudo's study in 2004 that researchers apparently asked themselves, "Why don't we look at the behavior of germ-free mice *without* stressing them out first, and just see if they are different to conventional animals?"—so suddenly opening the box on behavioral studies on germ-free mice.

How Do We Study the Brain and Behaviors in Mice?

Before we consider what the studies on behavior in germ-free mice showed, it might be interesting to consider what normal lab mice are like anyway, just in themselves. Because although lab mice are descended from wild-caught mice, they have been kept separate for so many generations now that they could be described almost as a separate species now, or at least as a separate subspecies.

However, lab mice are not even one homogenous group; there are numerous different strains, mainly descended from mice bred by mouse fanciers at the turn of the 19th century. By this time mouse fanciers had already been experimenting with breeding for several years in order to obtain different colored coats and various other characteristics.[11]

Mouse fanciers' mice and then lab mice quickly became very different from wild mice as a result of deliberate "back-breeding"—essentially getting siblings or other very closely related mice to mate. Of course, back-breeding led to very inbred strains, and, as we know, inbreeding can be deleterious and lead to the death of many animals. But scientists such as Clarence C. Little (1888–1971), an early mouse geneticist, working in the Harvard Bussey Institute, Massachusetts, were persistent. Between 1909 and 1911, Little recorded breeding 10,500 mice in an effort to obtain a totally inbred strain. Just one strain made it through, the first totally inbred genetically identical mouse strain in the world, the DBA (dilute brown agouti).

Today the DBA/2J strain is still used for research and is the oldest of all inbred strains. But there are over 450 other inbred strains now available, as well as many outbred strains (not genetically identical). Inbred strains are popular with scientists as they enable "consistent results." But scientists have to keep an eye on their mouse breeding. Only twenty generations of inbreeding are needed to obtain a strain potentially quite different from the one you started with. Given that mice can mature within six to eight weeks, on average live no longer than two years, and can have six babies every three weeks, this doesn't necessarily take very long.

Consequently, populations of lab mice since the turn of the century have exponentially increased. Jackson Labs, established in Maine in 1929 by C. C. Little, was already housing 25,000 mice by the time it was built. In 1947, when the lab suffered a terrible fire, over 90,000 mice died. Today in America, a conservative estimate of the number of lab mice is about 111 million; Jackson labs alone sell 3 million mice a year.[12]

Each of the most cited research teams working on the microbiome-gut-brain axis following Sudo's paper has used a different mouse strain, either inbred or outbred. Typical inbred strains include the BALB/c mice as used by Sudo and Swiss Websters (Neufeld).[13] Outbred strains include NMRI mice (Heijtz)[14] and NIH Swiss (Bercik).[15] Each strain has a characteristic phenotype, and each displays different personalities and idiosyncrasies, all exactly described and collected in a mouse phenotype database.[16]

To measure different phenotypes, rigorous batteries of tests have been developed over the years: first to assess simple things like eyesight and smell and whether the mice can move all four limbs properly, and then once these more basic parameters have been established, tests for intelligence, anxiety, or despair-like behavior are carried out. There would be no point checking a mouse for intelligence by using a maze, for example, if you didn't first know that its eyesight was intact.[17]

A clear description of a mouse phenotype also helps in the selection of the next generation. For example, in the generation of a mouse model for

ADHD, mice exhibiting high levels of "voluntary high wheel running" can be selected for breeding as a surrogate for hyperactivity.[18]

Some strains have well-known characters; for example, the BALB/c mice used in Sudo's study are considered to display a high level of anxiety-like behavior or "timidity." In contrast, the NIH Swiss mice used in Bercik's study are an outbred strain and exhibit less anxiety-like behavior and greater "boldness."[19]

There are a number of classic mouse tests used for testing anxiety-like behavior that get mentioned in each of these germ-free mouse behavioral studies, and it helps to be able to visualize what is going on. One of the most frequently mentioned is the Open Field Test (sometimes abbreviated to OF or OFT). It does not involve putting the mouse in a field. The mouse is simply put into a square tray to see what it does. This test is meant to simultaneously observe three parameters: general motor activity, exploratory behavior, and measures of anxiety—very ambitious for a tray. However, it seems to work. A timid mouse will stick to the edge, whereas a bolder mouse will go to the middle. Scientists measure the distance traveled by the mouse, the number of rearing occasions, and the amount of time spent in the middle compared to the edge. Of course, a scientist is no longer expected to sit on the edge of a work bench and peer over the edge of the tray to count rears and estimate distances traveled; it is all done automatically now using photobeams to disturb the animal as little as possible.

Another frequently mentioned test is the Elevated Plus Maze. This is a maze in the shape of a plus sign, raised high above the surface of the workbench. One line of the plus sign is relatively enclosed with high edges, the other is open. Mice prefer the safety of the enclosed arms, but they also like to explore the open arms. The Elevated Zero Maze is similar but better, in the shape of a perfect circle, again with two parts enclosed with high walls and with the advantage that the mice don't get stuck at one end of the plus sign. Both of these mazes are used as tests of anxiety-like behavior and were, in fact, used in early studies of certain anxiety medications such as benzodiazepines and antidepressants.[20]

So far, these tests have not been very mean. However, the last one that we will describe is a bit. The Forced Swimming Test involves first leaving them in a container of water completely out of their depth so that not even their long tail can touch the bottom, for fifteen minutes. The next day, they are put back for five minutes, and the time spent swimming versus floating is the parameter measured. If they float more than they swim, this is meant to be a high score for despair-like behavior. Some scientists note however, that this may well be a sensible learned response to the previous day's experience.

In Sudo's study, he doesn't mention measuring for anxiety-like or despair-like behavior. He simply "restrains" his mice to cause stress and then measures cortisol levels. Restraining a mouse is a well-recognized procedure used to cause acute stress in the mouse, and various parameters of stress reaction can then be measured. In this instance, restraining involves putting the mouse into a "well-ventilated" 5-centimeter-long tube and leaving it there for a certain measured amount of time. A smaller middle tube is then slipped over the tail to restrict movement even more.

If you can envisage a closed test tube lying on a bench and a mouse at one end of it with its tail sticking out through a hole in the end, then you will have a good picture of what a mouse looks like during a restraint test.[21] In Sudo's study, they were restrained like this for one hour, then their necks were broken to kill them, and a sample of blood taken straight out of their hearts to measure cortisol levels.

If you've never cared much about mice before (except for not liking them in your pantry cupboard and perhaps even killing them in a mousetrap on occasion), you may, all the same, be feeling a sense of unease about the way these mice are being used and bred in such huge numbers and in such an imperious way. It is well recognized that mice have not really entered into the collective consciousness of animal protection rights in the same way as larger animals.

On the plus side, there is a strong movement now for transparency in animal research, and many facilities offer a guided virtual tour online by the animal technicians so that anybody can see exactly how the animals live and are looked after in any one laboratory.

We have come a little off the topic of the microbiome and gut-brain axis here in order to find out a bit more about laboratory mice. But such large conclusions have been drawn about the effect of the gut microbiota on the brain from mouse studies that perhaps it is important to understand a bit about the mice themselves to see if these conclusions are reasonable or not. Even if the science and the conclusions drawn are secure, we would also need to consider how relevant any conclusions drawn from mice studies are to humans. Because, of course, we are not mice. We don't have ceca or have six babies every three weeks, and it is not natural or normal for us to display timidity and hide in boxes. Most of us are going out to work each day, not struggling to navigate a "maze" in the shape of a zero.

Although mice and humans are both mammals with certain similarities—especially at a cellular level, useful for scientists studying cancer, genetics, biochemistry, immunology, and many other important topics—it is obvious to all of us that mice and humans are very different when it comes to size, anatomy, and physiology. Simple comparisons of anatomy are found to be markedly different: the presence of a cecum in mice (vestigial in humans), physiology such as coprophagia (eating their own feces), and microanatomy (for example, the absence of a submucosa in the mouse colon). All of these differences have an effect on interpreting the presence of gut microbes and their actions.[22]

But to move from simple comparisons of anatomy to trying to draw parallels between mice and humans for complex and subtle parameters such as behavior, intelligence, mood disorders, or ADHD is fraught with difficulty and really not properly encapsulated by mouse models in which mice explore less or like running on a wheel more. It is extremely important not only to not anthropomorphize our microbes but also our mice. Avoiding exploring a maze does not show the mice are anxious but is only a very crude test to measure *anxiety-like behavior*. Although tests like these are reasonably well established and widely used, especially in pharmacology, they are also criticized by many scientists.

What Do Gut Microbiome-Gut-Brain Studies in Mice Show?

Now that we know a bit about lab mice, how their behavior is studied, and have an idea of the physiology of the gut-brain axis in all its power, let's go back to Sudo's paper and the mouse studies that he inspired. We now know he used inbred, germ-free mice of a constitutionally nervous strain

128 THE MICROBIOME

known as BALB/c . We know that he restrained twenty of these mice for one hour using the acute restraint equipment. He then killed them by breaking their necks, measured blood cortisol levels (a hormone that we now know is produced in the HPA axis), and compared the cortisol levels in these mice to a group of twenty BALB/c specific pathogen-free (SPF) mice (mice with a microbiome but no pathogens) and also two other groups of mice with just a single species of bacteria as their microbiome, either *E.coli* or a *Bifidobacterium.*

Following the restraint, the cortisol levels are a bit higher in the twenty germ-free mice than in the twenty SPF mice, but it's worth pointing out that the twenty mice with *E.coli* had levels higher still and that, in contrast, the mice with only *Bifidobacteria* had levels that were lower. Also no difference was seen at all between groups in the second phase of the trial, which we have not yet mentioned, where each group was subjected to an Ether Stress Test (exposure to an irritant chemical.) He does not mention any behavioral tests on any of these animals.

Nevertheless, he claims that the contradictory results from this tiny trial show that gut microbes alter the mouse brain's response to restraint stress. Over time, Sudo's study has been given a better and better outing. It is referenced on multiple occasions in both new studies and reviews, as here: "Microbes exert a major influence on both the HPA axis and on the immune system, compounding the link between the microbiota and the stress response. Sudo and colleagues were the first to demonstrate that germ-free mice who grew up in a sterile environment have an exaggerated HPA axis response to an acute stressor."[23]

A lot of conclusions to draw from one slightly raised cortisol test in twenty dead mice who had never been exposed to microbes until that morning, especially since the other stresser, ether, did not show any difference. Sudo's own (quite generous) conclusion that "commensal microbes affect the neural network" has progressed to microbes that "modulate" hormone levels[24] to microbes having "a major influence" on the HPA.

The assumption that the HPA is "hyperresponsive" or "exaggerated" is not borne out by comparing cortisol levels to parameters in other mouse studies measuring stress (see note 21), and the assertion that microbes exhibit a "major" influence on the HPA axis is not borne out by the overall normal development of germ-free animals.

Oddly, following Sudo's paper, there also seems to be a further assumption that germ-free animals are simply stressed in general. It is left to Neufeld to point out (in the usual hyperbolic terms) that although germ-free mice exhibited hyperresponsive HPA axis activity following stress as compared to SPF mice, "no associated behavioural changes were investigated in this study" (see note 13).

Neufeld's team took ten germ-free mice (Swiss Webster) out of their sterile environment and put them into an Open Field Test and Elevated Plus Maze and compared their behaviors with SPF mice. He found no difference in the Open Field Test; however, in the Elevated Plus Maze, germ-free mice appeared to exhibit *less* anxiety-like behavior. The same year, Heijtz's team tested only five mice (NMRI strain) in each group, but they ran the same tests and also said the germ-free mice displayed less anxiety-like behavior (see note 14). Following their lead, Sudo also turned to behavioral tests in a group of ten germ-free mice (BALB/c mice again), but in a show of one-upmanship performed them in a sterile environment and concluded that germ-free mice were more anxious.[25]

Consequently, various contradictory results have been found in subsequent small germ-free mouse studies, which, invoking Sudo's original paper, usually involve assessments of behavior, such as comparing germ-free to conventional mice as above, studying conventional mice treated with antibiotics, or studying the effect of administering probiotics. Studies have found in some cases that altered behavior is only found in male mice, others in both male and female, others that germ-free mice were more anxious, others that they are less anxious, some that probiotics reduced anxiety, others that antibiotics reduced anxiety, some that the vagus nerve had to be intact for this to work, others that cutting the vagus made no difference, some that colonizing the animals when young made them more anxious again, and others that colonizing when young made no difference (see note 24).

It is also typical in these studies to assume that any differences picked up in behavior between germ-free mice and conventional ones are due to the lack of microbes in the germ-free mice, rather than considering other possible causes such as the different mouse strains used, the different housing used for germ-free mice, and the constant noise of HEPA filters (high-efficiency particulate air filters), or indeed that the germ-free animal has had to be tested in a non-germ-free environment and is simultaneously coping with both the behavioral test and a massive onslaught of microbes.

Asking animal lab technicians today who work with germ-free mice whether the behavior of germ-free animals is any different, they say that they notice that the germ-free animals are calmer (but then because of their germ-free nature, they are interfered with less). They do note the pot-bellied appearance due to the enlarged cecum and also that the new pups are slightly slower to grow and are routinely left with their mothers for an extra two weeks before being separated.

How Could the Gut Microbiome Be Directing the Gut-Brain Axis?

One of the biggest problems of this field is "the difficulty of identifying causal pathways." In other words, if there really were two-way communication between the brain and the gut microbes, and microbes in the colon really were sending messages to our brain, then how would they do it?

The gut and the brain, as we know, communicate with each other with amazing finesse and detail, using both our conscious awareness of food, the food itself, as well as our unconscious sensing and control of the gut. It is well known that 95 percent of our digestion is completed in the small intestine, so how can signaling from microbes, principally located in the colon, fit in with all this? It is hard to imagine.

In Sudo's study on stress, the HPA axis is invoked, and his team makes a number of different suggestions to explain how gut microbes somehow communicate with the brain. One of the most mechanistic ideas, and perhaps the easiest one to visualize, is the suggestion that microbes somehow communicate with our brains via the vagus nerve. It's hard to know *how* this would happen, however scientists have found it straightforward to cut the vagus nerve in mice to see if it affected their results. They have obtained contradictory findings—some finding that it made a difference and others that it didn't.

Another potential route for gut microbes to communicate with the brain is by the production of inflammatory molecules. The different secretory cells in the lining of the gut are known to produce histamine, peptides, and many other chemicals, as we know, and it is possible that inflammatory molecules could trigger these cells to produce more of these chemicals. Microbes, especially pathogens, do trigger the immune system because they are infectious agents. That microbes can be seen as somehow being in charge of this mechanism and this could be called communicating with the gut-brain axis, however, is somewhat disingenuous.

However, another commonly cited mechanism, and perhaps the most persuasive, is via microbial metabolites. Perhaps microbes could be producing something, some potent chemical, or even a waste product, in large enough amounts to affect our well-being?

Do Microbial Metabolites Affect the Gut-Brain Axis?

Microbes, of course, produce plenty of potent chemicals inside us. They have to—they are living creatures like us. As well as all sorts of chemicals produced as part of their metabolism in order to stay alive, known as primary metabolites, they produce many other chemicals not directly necessary to their survival, known as secondary metabolites.

Microbial metabolites have interested scientists ever since the first one was identified in 1896 (mycophenolic acid), and this field is still an intensely fertile area of research, driven on by the battle to find the next antibiotic or the next cancer therapy.

To keep track of these microbial metabolites, there are various databases available; MiMeDB is one, listing over 55,000 different compounds, all made by microbes, most of which have been chemically exactly characterized with a known chemical structure.[26] Many have antibiotic properties, as, of course, microbes are in the business of survival and outcompeting their neighbors. Vancomycin, cyclosporin, tacrolimus, and lovastatin are all

132 THE MICROBIOME

examples of important microbial medicinal products used, respectively, as antibiotics, immunosuppressants, and cholesterol-lowering agents. Of the thousands of metabolites identified so far, approximately 150 are actively being used in medicine, industry, and agriculture. Those metabolites that don't appear to be active may still have a bioactivity somewhere but that hasn't been identified as yet.[27]

One of the most often mentioned groups of secondary metabolites produced by microbes in the gut—and probably the most voluminous—are the short-chain fatty acids (SCFAs) that we met in the last chapter. These are produced by gut bacteria whenever they digest or ferment the fiber in our guts. The commonest SCFAs are butyrate, propionate, and acetate, with these three together making over 95 percent of the total SCFA pool in our gut. The amount of SCFA that bacteria produce comes to a real and measurable amount, thought to be about 500–600 millimoles per day (based on fecal concentrations as a proxy of the production in the colon).

Most SCFAs are thought to be directly absorbed by colonocytes and used as energy. The tiny bit that remains is thought to be absorbed into the bloodstream and utilized by the liver, also as an energy substrate. Only a very minor fraction reaches other tissues, such as the brain, and the action, if any, of SCFAs on brain tissues is still unknown. Acetate and butyrate have been used in vitro to treat bits of brain in the lab to detect any influences on nerve cell growth or function, with indeterminate results so far.[28]

A medical team in Italy cut to the chase and simply dosed twenty-five obese children with one of these SCFAs, butyrate, giving a dose of 20 milligram/kilogram to each child once a day for six months, to see if it would affect their appetite. This experiment shows a certain amount of chutzpa. It simply looks to see if butyrate, a bacterial metabolite or "postbiotic," does anything, and it uses a significant dosage. However, it seems to have caused minimal harm to the children: transient mild nausea and headache in just two and a very slight effect on weight loss in the treatment group.[29]

Some scientists have gone as far as suggesting that some bacterial metabolites could be actual "neurotransmitters." However, the direct production of a neurotransmitter by an enteric bacterial species has not been described. Typically, microbes don't tend to make the same secondary metabolites as higher plants or animals (see note 27).

If a bacterial microbe could directly produce a human neurotransmitter, this metabolite would obviously not be a neurotransmitter for the microbe. Even if this molecule could then cross our gut barrier, blood-brain barrier, and nerve barriers, it would still not meet the criteria for being a neurotransmitter, as to meet this definition, neurotransmitters have to be released in a nerve synapse in response to presynaptic depolarization (see note 19).

Can Microbes Affect Depression?

The fact that microbes can't directly make neurotransmitters hasn't stopped researchers really zooming in on one particular human chemical: serotonin. As we already know, serotonin is a key neurotransmitter for the gut, and some is also found in the brain. One well-established biochemical model of depression suggests that the reason people have low mood is because they don't have enough serotonin. In support of this theory, medication that increases serotonin levels improves depression symptoms. Selective serotonin reuptake inhibitor (SSRI) medications, such as the familiar Prozac (fluoxetine), are thought to work in this way.

Although microbes can't make serotonin themselves, there is plenty of discussion as to whether microbes could somehow activate certain cells that do make serotonin and affect the brain in this way. For example, could gut microbes produce metabolites that chemically activate the enterochromaffin cells in the gut to produce more serotonin? Enterochromaffin cells are activated by both chemical and neurological stimuli in the gut-brain axis and even by the physical presence of food, but it is possible that the presence of microbes could contribute as well.

There is some evidence in vitro to suggest that the presence of microbes does affect serotonin production, although no specific metabolite has been identified. As usual, the case has been slightly overstated, and instead of saying, microbes "may slightly affect the production of serotonin from enterochromaffin cells," the authors announce that "gut microbiota regulate host serotonin biosynthesis."[30]

134 THE MICROBIOME

An alternative approach to detecting the effect of the gut microbes on the brain has been to measure the serum levels of neurotransmitters and the amino acids needed to produce them in both germ-free and conventional animals. There does appear to be a difference. Serum levels of tryptophan, an essential amino acid needed to form serotonin tend to be 40 to 60 percent lower in conventional animals compared to germ-free. But when serum serotonin is compared, levels are two to three times *higher* in conventional animals.[31]

Rather than looking for a microbiome-gut-brain axis style of explanation where the gut microbes are "controlling" the levels of serotonin production, a more likely reason is that the higher serum levels of tryptophan in germ-free animals is because they have the full benefit of their digestive enzymes and thus a more efficient absorption. But why serotonin levels are lower and what this means for the animal is harder to interpret.

These comparisons do show, though, that the presence of microbes in the gut potentially has an effect on the production of neurotransmitters and perhaps even the function of the gut and the brain—but not in a hyperbolic "microbes are controlling us" kind of way. It is simply that when gut bacteria are present, they just happen to degrade our digestive enzymes, which means that as a species we have had to adapt and make more digestive enzymes to compensate. Germ-free animals then end up with more digestive enzymes than they need. In this explanation, bacteria are not controlling or directing us, but it is clear that the absence of these metabolic processes in germ-free animals may have affected the absorption of certain essential amino acids.

The funny thing is that with all this discussion of whether bacteria are "controlling" or deliberately increasing our serotonin levels, it turns out that antidepressant SSRI medications are antibacterial and therefore harmful to the microbiome. Patients who are on SSRIs for depression and who have higher serotonin levels both in the gut and the brain often have major disruption of their gut microbiomes as a result of this medication.

In conclusion, according to reviews in the microbiome field, "there remains healthy scepticism as to whether recent work may have translational potential for treating anxiety and depression in humans" (see note 24), and in almost the same phrase a few years later, "there remains much healthy scepticism in the field as to whether such findings in animals have any implications for human mental health."[32]

You could argue that these remarks are rather generous because there also remains a lot of healthy skepticism about the microbiome-gut-brain field in general, even when just referring to mice. It is a scientific area of research where over 50 percent of publications are reviews. Trying to make sense of small, contradictory, behavioral mouse trials—where even the most cited papers contain evidence that is, at best, "suggestive," is certainly challenging, especially considering that more than a quarter of articles and reviews on the "microbiota-gut-brain" are published by just one team.[33]

Could Microbes Have Evolved to Affect the Gut-Brain Axis?

Could microbes in the gut have evolved to manipulate the brain to ensure their own survival? It seems farfetched. However, we have all heard that horrible story of the fungi that hijacks ants and makes them climb high up in the canopy and finally bite on vegetation before they die, anchoring the ant at a high elevation and enabling efficient fungal sporulation. Could bacteria be doing this to us and controlling us in this way? Could they be telling us to eat certain foods for their own benefit, as the headlines in the newspapers have implied? The short answer is no. It is obvious to an evolutionary geneticist based on the one thing we know about gut microbes, their variability, that this is impossible.

Microbes can affect host behavior for their own ends, as in the ant example, and we principally know this from parasite infections, but examples like this are surprisingly rare and difficult to prove. Not that microbes don't affect our behavior; this happens all the time. For example, when we have an infection and get a fever and want to lie down, here it is our immune system fighting off the infection that gives us symptoms such as fever and tiredness and makes us want to rest. It is the second part that is hard to prove: that the altered behavior increases the fitness and survival of the microbe.

In the case of a gut microbiome, if we imagine a particular gut microbe somehow persuading us to eat a certain food (perhaps by making a special metabolite), we could then further imagine that this food would increase the chance of the microbe's survival. However, it is clear that the microbe would have to put energy into making the special metabolite. If we consider further and visualize all of the other species of microbes in the gut that are living next to our particular microbe, then we can see that they would be competing with each other for survival. It is clear that microbes that are only using their energy to reproduce and grow and not investing energy in a special metabolite will reproduce more successfully. They may even benefit from the additional food even though they themselves have not invested any energy into obtaining it.

It is clear that the other microbial species, investing only in reproducing, will rapidly out-compete the microbe making the special metabolite. This particular gut microbe is likely to be rapidly lost in the face of the competition; it would be surprising indeed if it lasted more than a few microbial generations.

It is this variability of our gut microbiome that points us away from any special connection or evolution with one kind of bacteria. We can be absolutely confident that no one bacterium controls our thoughts (or our appetite), and it is very unlikely that there is any one bacterium causing depression or protecting us from it.[34]

However, just because one single microbe is not manipulating us doesn't mean the presence of microbes is not affecting us at all. It might be, as we have discussed, that some kind of general waste product from bacteria could affect us in some way, like the SCFA (although as we have seen, they don't seem to particularly, even in large doses) or the way bacteria deactivate bile acids, which then affects the absorption of various nutrients and essential amino acids, as in the case of tryptophan.

It may be that we would be calmer without a microbiome—as some report germ-free mice appear to be—or perhaps we would be more anxious as others have reported, or maybe it would make no difference to our behavior at all; after all we only have contradictory reports of small numbers of lab-bred, inbred, germ-free mice to go on. But whether gut microbes affect our brain or not, it is clear that our gut-brain axis is absolutely a real phenomenon—a complex, fast-acting set of reflexes that can act fully independently of any microbial input.

At the end of the day, humans will never be without microbes. We have evolved to cope with the large variety of microbes inside us, and these certainly digest our bile acids, ferment our foods, and make waste products such as SCFA. Our bodies have learned to compensate for this so that we still produce the right amount of bile acids, absorb the right amount of amino acids, and make the right amount of neurotransmitters in spite of their presence.

And finally, with regard to future communication about this fascinating topic, we don't need the links between the microbiome and the gut-brain axis to be overstated.[35] Exact and clear communication about the effect of the microbiome on our bodies will help our understanding of this topic much better than runaway statements about microbes, diet, and what it means to be human, because the way microbes have clearly affected our evolution, our immune system, and our nutrient absorption is fascinating enough.

7

THE MICROBIOME AND THE GENITALS

Why Are the Microbes of the Genital Tract Important?

The microbes of the genital tract, particularly the female genital tract, have a particular importance to our health, and even our survival. This is because of the close proximity the vaginal microbes have to the uterus. Research on the vaginal microbiome has a long history, and in keeping with the other microbiomes we have discussed, the reason for this wasn't just curiosity, but a life-threatening medical issue. Just as with the skin microbiome, where the concern was with handwashing and surgical wound infections, and the neonatal gut microbiome, where the issue was infant survival, research on the vaginal microbiome also began because of a serious medical issue: uterine infections following childbirth. An infection of the womb following birth could in the past—and even today—lead to the new mother becoming very seriously ill or even dying.

By talking about infections of the womb, it may seem as if we are straying from the topic of microbiomes into the topic of infectious disease. It is true that the cause of endometritis (womb infections), or as it is properly known, post-puerperal infection, is now well understood to be due to certain pathogenic bacteria. But at the start of research on the vaginal microbiome in the 1880s, there were still many unknowns. Was it a microbe causing post-puerperal infections, and if so, which one? And if it was a microbe, where had it come from? Some doctors thought that any infection of the womb always came from outside of the mother, for example, from the doctor's or midwife's hands during a vaginal examination. Other doctors argued that as there were so many bacteria already in the vagina, infections of the womb must come from the woman herself, the doctrine of "autoinfection." In the late 19th century, this wasn't just a question or a discussion; there was a real row among medical men about the concept of "autoinfection" versus external infection.

What Was the Importance of Aseptic Technique When It Came to Childbirth?

The importance of handwashing had, of course, first been brought to the world's attention by poor Ignaz Philipp Semmelweis (1818–1865), a physician working in Vienna. Semmelweis instituted handwashing at the Vienna General Hospital's First Obstetrical Clinic, bringing down maternal death rates from a horrifying 18 percent to the greatly improved (but still more than twenty times today's figures) 2 percent. Although ignored and ridiculed at the time, his work has never been forgotten since and is always cited in discussions of post-puerperal infection, whether it be a journal article written in 1870 or a paper published today.

It was well accepted by this time, as is easily ascertained by reading the medical textbooks of the day, that handwashing or hand sterilization before performing a vaginal examination was seen as absolutely imperative (see Figure 7.1). In *A System of Obstetrics by American Authors*, a obstetrics textbook published in 1888, the authors advise, "A thorough scrubbing of the hands with brush and soap, followed by a washing in the bichloride solution of 1 : 1000." This instruction is followed by extensive quotes of maternal mortality rates from different medical centers following the adoption of hand sterilization, as each center began to see marked improvements to the maternal death rate. These changes were probably happening within the author's working lifetime: it is noted that the death rate during or following pregnancy dropped from 10 percent in the 1860s to 1.1 percent or even 0.3 percent by the 1870s.

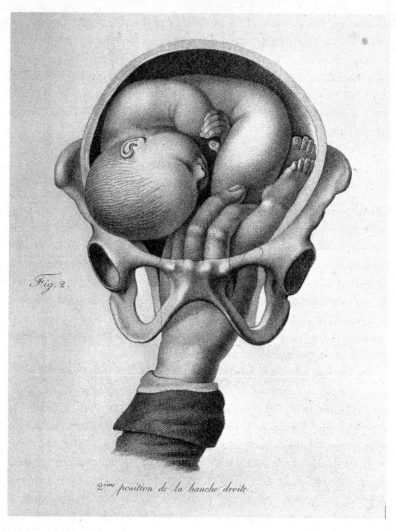

Figure 7.1 This French engraving from 1825 shows a vaginal examination in which the caregiver is grasping the knee of a fetus to pull it down so that it can be delivered feet first.

Journals in the 1880s repeatedly point out that this cleanliness does not just apply to the obstetrician but to the woman's genital areas and the room she is being examined in as well. "The maternal parts should be rinsed in a solution of creolin. Aseptic towels should be pinned around the thighs and over the mons. The patient is now ready for an internal examination, which should be repeated as seldom as possible."[1]

The antiseptic solutions at this time are nerve-rackingly different from the ones we would use now. Here, a family doctor attending home births describes his routine: "I always wash my hands thoroughly in warm water and soap, then dip them in a solution of carbolic acid (1 in 40) and dry them. When making an examination, I smear the examining finger and whole right hand with antiseptic Vaseline (1 in 1,000 perchloride of mercury)."[2]

But despite this emphasis on handwashing, when there was a death due to sepsis—and there were still many—there must have been a lot of harsh words directed at the attending health workers, whether doctors or midwives, implying that the clinician involved had not followed antiseptic precautions properly.

The concept of "autoinfection," that the offending microbe was already in the woman's vagina, implied that it was not the obstetrician's fault if she became ill or died and was a good get-out clause. Indeed, there really were cases where labor had gone smoothly, no vaginal examination had been attempted, and yet the woman had still died of a womb infection. At this time, no one was really sure whether it was even a microbe causing the fever, let alone which microbe it was or where it had come from.

You may be thinking to yourself, "Why 'he'?" or "Why medical 'men'?"—but the reason for this is simple: at this time, most doctors were men. It was usual for doctors to vote against the admission of women into medical courses, and even if trained, women were often not allowed to graduate. Men were the ones working as obstetricians and writing in the journals, and it was men who drove the medical agenda.

Because of this, there is a sense of inequality in ownership of this topic; researchers are mainly male, and the patients are all female, seemingly passive recipients of advice, examinations, and interventions, and often in extremis during these times, in labor or sick with post-puerperal sepsis. It's deeply distressing to think of the deaths of these young women, summed up so brusquely in the improving maternal mortality rates of the various hospitals at the time.

On the other hand, those mainly male doctors and bacteriologists are often deeply concerned about maternal death rates from sepsis; some are even obsessed with the topic and come back to it again and again in the journals of the time.

What Did Early Research on the Vaginal Microbiome Show?

Dr. Albert Doderlein (1860–1941), an obstetrician in Germany, was one of the earliest and most scientific researchers on the vaginal microbiome and also the most influential. When he wrote his first paper on this topic, he was still an assistant obstetrician at the Trier Institute of Midwifery in Leipzig. Published in 1887, here he is simply trying to associate any fever in a woman who has just given birth with a change in the microbes of her vagina. You can tell he is very junior at this time, as at the end he gives his "sincerest thanks at this point for your lovely welcome and varied suggestions in carrying out these investigations" to the director of the hygienic institute, Professor Hofman.[3]

During his introduction, he notes that even with strict antiseptic guidance and handwashing, institutions that allow additional internal examinations by students practicing their technique have a mortality rate of 1.9 percent, whereas those that do not have a mortality rate of 0.56 percent. Examining women during childbirth, even antiseptically, was increasing the rate of mortality by 400 percent.

Either the disinfection had to be even stricter or, if disinfection couldn't do any more than it already had, then internal examinations had to be limited to the utmost. Indeed, when epidemic puerperal infections were raging, internal examinations were already banned altogether, an action supported by ministerial decree in Prussia.

Doderlein plunges straight into the autoinfection debate. "Self-infection refers to an infection for which the doctor or midwife cannot be held responsible. It is statistically proven that such cases occur."

That it was usual for the vagina to contain a variety of bacteria was well known at the time. "The vaginal secretion always contains cleavage fungi (bacteria) of various kinds. The microscopic examination already convinces us of this. It contains bacteria and cocci in countless quantities in every pregnant woman and mother." But as usual, trying to identify the microbial cause of post-puerperal sepsis was made much more difficult by the presence of the microbiome. This is in contrast say to identifying the microbes causing a blood infection, where, because the blood is sterile, there is no difficulty in identifying the microbe responsible.

Doderlein, as well as acknowledging the presence of these varied and numerous bacilli, also asks—just as we did when discussing both the skin and gut microbiome—how did all of these bacteria get into the vagina in the first place? He does not shy away from discussing intimate details: "The first thing to take into account is the penis. Bacilli have been detected in the preputial secretion, the smegma . . . and there is no question that it can occasionally introduce other pathogenic germs in addition to gonorrhea, syphilis, and tubercle (TB) germs." We will come back to the microbiome of the penis later in the chapter.

He points out the close proximity of the anus to the vagina, which would easily allow transmission of fecal bacteria. He suggests that the woman's own fingers might be an agent of transmission or "possibly foreign bodies being introduced." Perhaps he is thinking here of tampons or pads used by the women themselves during their periods.

He is critical of other researchers' sloppy approaches to obtaining samples from the vagina and describes his own sterile technique in detail. By the end of this paper (after a lot of mention of the different "seamstresses" that seemed to have been his patients), he concludes, firstly, that under normal conditions the healthy uterus is sterile; secondly, that if virulent streptococci are found in the uterus, they are associated with the development of fever; and finally that the vagina contains countless "germs" of all kinds, *including* pathogens.

However, it was his 1892 paper that really transformed the field. Titled "The Vaginal Secretion and Its Significance for Puerperal Fever," he was the first to really focus on the microbes found in the vagina and try to identify both which ones they were and what they do.

What Does Vaginal Discharge Consist Of?

To start with, Doderlein analyzed vaginal discharge. It is still agreed today that vaginal discharge is formed, as he described, from both cervical mucus secreted by the glandular cells on the cervix and serous fluid (the watery component of blood) simply exuding from the vaginal walls. The cells lining the vagina include no glandular cells. As well, vaginal discharge also contains superficial epithelial cells shed from the vagina and, of course, all of the bacilli that we will come to shortly.

Having analyzed the content of vaginal discharge, Doderlein decided to measure the amount of vaginal discharge. He did this by rinsing the area with warm water and collecting the resulting fluid. Who he managed to convince to have her vagina rinsed and how he managed to persuade them is unknown, but the result is still quoted in modern textbooks today (0.5–0.8 grams), as presumably, scientists don't care (or don't dare) to repeat the procedure. He then ascertained that although the cervical mucous is alkaline overall, the vaginal discharge is acidic with a pH of 4.5. Using the chemical methods of the day, he showed that the acid was formed of lactic acid.

Which Microbes Are in the Vaginal Microbiome?

To analyze the bacteria present, Doderlein next examined smears under a microscope. Just like Escherich when studying neonatal stools, he found that vaginal smears were dominated by just one microbe: hundreds and thousands of them (see Figure 7.2).

These microbes were difficult to grow—culture after culture grew nothing at all. But when he finally succeeded, he describes a non-sporing, non-motile bacillus that preferred to be kept moist, grew best at blood temperature on a special agar, and needed an atmosphere with reduced amounts of oxygen. He worked out that it was this bacterium that kept the pH of vaginal discharge low by making lactic acid, the very same acid he had already identified, and called it "vaginal bacillus."

His paper was so influential that although this bacterium was initially referred to as "vaginal bacillus," it soon became known as "Doderlein's bacillus," a term still used today in some reference materials. Eventually renamed *Lactobacillus acidophilus*, it was later realized that this species was,

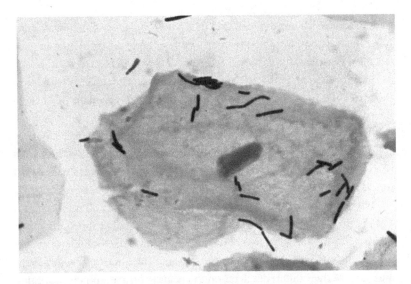

Figure 7.2 This Gram-stained photomicrograph of a vaginal smear specimen reveals the presence of a squamous epithelial cell 60–100 micrometers across, and numerous Gram-positive bacilli, or rod-shaped bacteria, likely lactobacilli, each 10–15 micrometers long.

in fact, a *group* of closely related species. We will come back to this later in the chapter.

The number of these lactobacilli in healthy vaginal discharge was enormous, accounting for over 95 percent of the bacteria present. But to Doderlein this was baffling. How could this be? The vagina, as we have already described, is absolutely not a sterile area. Where then were all the other bacteria, introduced from stool, from tampons, from sexual intercourse? How was it possible for just one bacterium to dominate even though so many different bacteria were constantly being introduced?

What Do the Microbes in the Vaginal Microbiome Do?

Doderlein thought that perhaps somehow these lactobacilli stopped other bacteria from growing. This important concept of "colonization resistance" is one that we have already come across both in the skin chapter with regard to *Staphylococcus epidermidis* and the neonatal chapter in reference to bifidobacteria. To test the idea that the lactobacilli were somehow keeping other bacteria out, he plated them out on agar and added colonies of what he called "virulent streptococci." Streptococcal growth was clearly inhibited as they grew closer to the established colonies of lactobacilli. It wasn't just the acid conditions that the lactobacilli engendered, although this helped (he checked for this). It was the lactobacilli themselves.

To prove the theory that the lactobacilli kept the other bacteria out beyond doubt, he then infused a sample of *Staphylococcus aureus* into the vagina of a virgin (some of us may be thinking this really is a step too far) to see what would happen. The *S. aureus* was undetectable within a few days.

His research was not just based on a few patients but on samples from 194 pregnant women. As he continued to study smear after smear under the microscope, he started to spot different patterns in the sets of microbes that he found. Naturally, he began to try to group these into different groups and analyze their different effects on the health of these women, work that is still being refined today.

He noted that 55 percent of his patients had vaginal secretions dominated by lactobacilli, in his view an indication of a normal discharge. Another group of women, also healthy, had a "richer" set of microbes, with more variety and more species but still no pathogens, and these accounted for 35.5 percent. Because neither of these groups had pathogens present, he felt that it would be safe to perform a vaginal examination during labor in these women, if an aseptic technique was used.

In the remaining 9 percent, he identified "virulent streptococci." These were the women he was concerned about. Although these bacteria usually caused no problems to these women's health, if they were examined—even with aseptic techniques—the virulent streptococci could be pushed into the wrong place, up into the uterus, and then cause a womb infection. In his view, the risk of autoinfection in these women was high.

His research was quoted extensively and discussed everywhere. William E Ground, an obstetrician writing in America in 1894 (who could either read German or had a good translation), passes the key points of Doderlein's paper on to his audience: the acidic nature of vaginal discharge, the "vaginal bacillus" (he uses this term), and its colonization resistance.

However, he stridently disagrees with Doderlein about what he calls "the absurd and meaningless term autoinfection." In his view, this term had no place in a scientific discussion. The concept was a myth, and the occurrence of puerperal sepsis "prima facie evidence that pathogenic germs have at some time gained admission to the maternal parts from without." Ground allows that it doesn't always have to be from the surgeon. The sources of infection, in his view and in order of importance are first the midwife or attending nurse, second the surgeon, and third the husband or the patient herself.

Although Ground has put the attending clinicians first as the source of these lethal infections, he is brutal in his description of the husband. "Most men touch their penis several times a day while urinating, and yet I dare say few of them ever think of washing it, no matter how dirty their occupations, before thrusting it into the parturient canal at night."

Do Microbes from the Vaginal Microbiome Cause Post-Puerperal Infection?

It took several more decades and the development of new microbial techniques to sort out this question. In the meantime, obstetricians had to push on with the two key approaches to reducing post-puerperal infection already identified: a thorough aseptic technique and keeping vaginal examinations to a minimum.

But in the 1930s, Rebecca Lancefield (1895–1981), a bacteriologist working in New York, developed a method to further differentiate those virulent streptococcal bacteria so frequently mentioned by Doderlein. Following her work, it was recognized there were over 30 or more different types of streptococci, some of them worse than others.

The scene now moves to Queen Charlotte's Obstetric Hospital in London, England, where Leonard Colebrook (1883–1967) and his sister Dora Colebrook (1884–1965), both bacteriologists, were working. Using Lancefield's new techniques, the Colebrooks finally proved that the streptococci found in normal vaginal discharge in healthy pregnant women were *not* the ones causing sepsis. The really pathogenic bacterium, the one that caused the lethal post-puerperal epidemics of the 19th century, was Lancefield

148 THE MICROBIOME

Group A streptococcus, now known as *Streptococci pyogenes*. It almost always came from an outside source. The normal microbes of the vaginal microbiome almost never cause a post-puerperal infection.

However, although the Colebrooks had finally proved that *Streptococci pyogenes* was absolutely not part of the vaginal microbiome, some doctors were reluctant to give up the concept of autoinfection, a concept now known (in that typical evolution of terms) as "endogenous puerperal infection." As L. Colebrook points out in his typical hard-hitting way, "I know that that conception is dear to the heart of some obstetricians, and they will not readily part with it."

But the Colebrooks were unrelenting. They worked not just on identifying the correct species from any unwell patient with post-puerperal sepsis that came into their hospital (and they had plenty) but also on identifying the exact *strain* of each sample that they obtained. They did this in order to trace the source of each and every infection from every woman who succumbed to this infection. By taking vaginal swabs from each patient and comparing them with nasal swabs from anyone who had been in contact with her—her nurse, her midwife, her obstetrician, her partner, her family, even her children—they could work out exactly who the lethal infection had come from. Of the forty-eight infected patients that they studied, six had caught it from their own throats, twenty-four had caught it from a midwife or doctor, and nine had caught it from either their husband or children. In the remainder, a source was not identified.[4]

L. Colebrook's research was not just theoretical. His friend's wife died of this condition in the same year his paper was published. Young and healthy, she had given birth easily but developed a fever on the third day and tragically died sixteen days later. Like an inexorable detective from a 1930s murder-mystery novel, so popular at the time, Colebrook went from contact to contact, taking swabs in his role as both friend and bacteriologist. Finally, like a terrifying Judge Dredd, he identified a matching strain on the throat swab of the assisting nurse. This nurse, who had not worn a mask while nursing the patient, had come straight from temporary duty in the children's ward of a small hospital where there were cases of tonsillitis. We can only imagine how devastating it would be to know you were responsible for the death of a patient in this way.[5]

Colebrook focuses adamantly on preventing further cases. To have identified the nurse as responsible simply means that he can prevent her from spreading it to yet more patients.

He is the only one to acknowledge how hard and how boring this constant attention to hygiene was. "Antisepsis care adds enormously to the tedious routine and the expense of maternity work." He did not expect to eradicate maternal deaths from sepsis altogether, but his dearest wish was to decrease the maternal death rate to 0.2 percent, which in his view would be achievable with the routine use of gloves, masks, and regular swabs of medical attenders.

But not long after this, L. Colebrook was the first to use a novel chemotherapy agent to treat a case of post-puerperal infection, a medication called Prontosil. Since those first triumphant lifesaving antibiotics were used, the emphasis on which healthcare worker (or husband or child) is responsible for an infection has receded. Prompt treatment with antibiotics for post-puerperal infection is still absolutely essential, but regular swabbing of medical staff has never caught on.

Are Vaginal Examinations in Pregnancy Still a Recognized Cause of Infections?

In modern obstetric guidelines, the importance of handwashing and sterility during childbirth is presumed so obvious that it is simply not mentioned. In contrast to the pages and pages on aseptic technique in 19th-century obstetrics textbooks, there are literally no chapters on it at all in a modern obstetrics textbook. Aseptic techniques are simply known as "standard infection prevention and control." This includes ordinary hand hygiene (just as we described in the dermatology chapter), gloves, aseptic surgical techniques, clean equipment, and skin antisepsis—all absolutely standard.

But in spite of access to "standard infection prevention and control," the 19th-century approach of keeping vaginal examinations to a minimum is still followed. No matter how good the technique or how aseptic the

150 THE MICROBIOME

approach, it is recognized that there is always a chance of introducing infection. During pregnancy, vaginal examinations are typically avoided, and external examinations only are used to check mother and baby. Once in labor, a vaginal examination is recommended at the outset to check what stage of labor the woman has reached, but after that no more frequently than once every four hours. The widely cited World Health Organization (WHO) guidelines strongly advise that "priority must be given to restricting the frequency and total number of vaginal examinations. This is particularly crucial in situations where there are other risk factors for infection. Multiple vaginal examinations are recognised contributors to infectious morbidities."

Unfortunately, WHO advice is not always followed. A recent study found that women in some countries are physically and verbally abused during labor, and of those experiencing a vaginal examination, up to 60 percent had not consented. A potential excess of vaginal examinations, regarded as five or more per labor, is also not uncommon and is seen in over a third of women in some settings. Despite WHO's efforts to improve labor management and the availability of antibiotics, maternal mortality remains an ever-present reality for many women.[6,7]

Are Lactobacilli Still Regarded as a Key Vaginal Microbe Today?

Because of these risks of infection, research on pregnant women has been avoided for many years and regarded almost as taboo by some scientists. Focus instead has switched to women who are not pregnant, usually separated into three groups: pre-pubertal girls, post-menopausal older women, and the group in between who are not pre-pubertal, pregnant, or post-menopausal but typically having regular periods and approximately between the ages of thirteen and fifty-two. This group is sometimes known by the cumbersome title of post-menarcheal/pre-menopausal (PMPM) females, but essentially, we mean potentially fertile women.

To begin with, early researchers simply wanted to confirm Doderlein's findings and identify the presence of the same vaginal bacilli as he had.

The Microbiome and the Genitals   151

However, it was difficult to be sure which species Doderlein had been referring to. The various lactic acid bacilli were sometimes hard to differentiate, having similar growing conditions and biochemical reactions, as well as all making lactic acid. But when grown next to each other, it was possible to detect subtle differences in colony appearance and biochemical reactions— not only between Doderlein's bacillus, bifidobacteria, and *Lactobacillus acidophilus*, but also *within* the colonies of Doderlein's bacilli. This led bacteriologists to suggest that "Doderlein's bacillus forms a heterogenous group," and in 1931, the presence of three different strains was suggested.[8]

In spite of this, for many years, vaginal bacilli were still known as *Lactobacilli acidophilus*, and in some countries, ordinary live yogurt was thought to be a perfectly adequate way of treating certain vaginal conditions. It was only in 1980, using early DNA sequencing techniques, that this very closely related group of bacilli was found to encompass five different lactobacilli species: *L. crispatus*, *L. amylovorus*, *L. gallinarum*, *L. gasseri*, and *L. johnsonii*, and finally differentiated from the quite different yogurt species *Lactobacilli acidophilus*.[9] A further additional lactobacillus species, *L. iners*, obtained from a woman in Sweden, was detected in 1999, and others have since been described.[10]

Once identified, these bacilli have been found to be ubiquitous, found in human females all over the world—from Europe to America, from Africa to Asia, and from China to Japan—implying a very strong co-evolutionary connection between us and these bacilli and an evolutionary advantage to having them, just like the bifidobacteria in new babies.

Unlike some of the other microbiomes we have looked at so far, a healthy vaginal microbiome in humans appears to be one with hardly any species at all. The less diverse the vaginal microbiome is, the healthier it appears to be; this is in stark contrast to the gut, where the more diverse, the better. In the vaginal microbiome, usually only ten to fifteen species are found in any one person, and each microbiome is typically dominated by just one lactobacilli species.

Because of this, the vaginal microbiome is, at first glance, much easier to get to grips with than other, more variable microbiomes, and the

152 THE MICROBIOME

focus on just one species gives a feeling of clarity and elegance to vaginal microbiome research and a pleasant impression of building on previous knowledge.

Of course, there is still plenty of variability to observe. As we know, the microbes in any one microbiome can never be static; at any one time, they are reproducing, dying, and being incessantly cleared by our body's innate immune defenses. In particular, variability in the vaginal microbiome is linked to levels of estrogen. This is because the cells in the vagina that make glycogen, the lactobacilli's key substrate, are very responsive to hormonal changes. The more estrogen there is, the more glycogen these cells make, and the more lactobacilli are therefore present. During menstruation, when estrogen levels drop, the number of lactobacilli also tend to decrease, and during the midcycle, when estrogen levels rise again, there is a corresponding increase in glycogen, and this allows the number of lactobacilli to bounce back.

Do All Women Have Lactobacilli?

Although there is a cyclical variation of lactobacilli coming and going according to the menstrual cycle, in fact not all women have a vaginal microbiome containing lactobacilli. Some women have a different, more varied set of microbes, as originally identified by Doderlein. But does this matter?

It has been shown that a vaginal microbiome dominated by lactobacilli really does appear to protect women from genital infections, just as Doderlein thought. Not just during pregnancy but also during day-to-day life and particularly on exposure to sexually transmitted diseases (STDs). As well as being proved in vitro for a wide range of pathogens, this effect has also been established in vivo by observing higher rates of STD infection in women without lactobacilli compared to women with lactobacilli. This effect applies to all sorts of pathogens, ranging from yeast infections to gonorrhea, chlamydia, syphilis, *Trichomonas vaginalis*, and even viral infections such as genital herpes and genital warts, with a rate of infections approximately three times higher in those without lactobacilli compared to those with.

But even if a woman did get one of these infections, with the availability of modern clinics, she can easily be treated, and so over time, interest in the protective effects of lactobacilli waned. However, with the advent of HIV in the 1980s, interest reawakened, and once again lactobacilli were seen as important. Many women at the time were being encouraged to use a spermicide or microbicides vaginally to reduce the chances both of catching HIV and of getting pregnant. But then researchers became aware that spermicide might inadvertently be disrupting the lactobacilli and increasing the rates of STD in these women and concerns about the loss of the protective effects of lactobacilli were raised once again. By the late 1990s, highly active anti-retroviral treatment (HART) to treat HIV had been developed and, just as before, once an effective chemotherapy had been established, the need for and interest in the protective effects of lactobacilli receded.[11]

Research in the vaginal microbiome has, of course, continued, with the focus shifting away from post-puerperal infections, STDs, and HIV to unsolved clinical issues such as infertility, prematurity, and infections in newborns. If different sorts of vaginal microbiomes could just be categorized in more detail, perhaps researchers might be able to associate a certain sort of microbiome with something meaningful such as a community, a country, or a clinically important health issue.

Community state types (CST), a new way of categorizing vaginal microbiomes into groups, were developed exactly for this purpose. Based on 396 asymptomatic women and published in 2011 by a scientist named J. Ravel working in France, five different CST groups are described, from Group I to V.

Group I was dominated by *L. crispatus* and found in 26 percent of women; Group II by *L. gasseri* (6.3 percent); Group III by *L. iners* (34.1 percent); and Group V by *L. jensenii*. Group IV has no or minimal lactobacilli presence and a much more heterogeneous set of microbes, including anaerobic bacteria such as *Prevotella*, *Gardnerella*, *Eggerthella*, and others.[12]

Having identified these groups, Ravel was now in a position to comment on which group was common in which community, or which lactobacilli appeared to be the best in some way. *L. cripsatus* in Group I had the lowest pH of the lactobacilli, at 4.0, long thought to be a mark of health. The more variable Group IV had the highest pH, at 5.3.[13]

154   THE MICROBIOME

Research on individual lactobacilli species and their association with good or ill health is still thought to have great potential, with *L. iners* in Group III identified as perhaps the least beneficial and most unstable of the lactobacilli species so far. CST Group IV, the variable one, is also frequently singled out for special attention. It is important to note that the microbes present in this group are also known for their lactic acid–producing abilities and that all of the women analyzed in this trial were healthy. However, concerns that Group IV may be associated with a higher risk of contracting sexually transmitted infections if exposed still remain.

The implications of belonging to Group IV, or indeed any of the groups, are hard to interpret because it turns out the CST groups are not stable. They are based on a snapshot, a cross-section of women's microbiomes, captured for a single moment in time. If we do a temporal study, taking swabs from each woman say, twice a week, (and Ravel went on to do just that), it turns out that most women aren't just in one CST group but are always changing from one to another group.

Further studies show that many women don't really fit into any CST group but are somewhere in between, indicating that perhaps CSTs, although convenient to visualize, are not real or distinct groups but rather better imagined as a continuum, with women switching unconsciously from one to another according to what is happening in their life at the time.[14]

Which Lifestyle Factors Can Affect the Composition of the Vaginal Microbiome?

A new scientific approach known as "citizen science" has shed more light on this variability recently by allowing the subjects themselves to be involved in the research. The citizen science ISALA study (named after the first female doctor in Belgium) somehow captured the public's attention, and a self-taken vaginal swab and ninety-minute survey was undertaken by over 3,000 participants from throughout Belgium, with some households so keen to participate that women from three generations (aged eighteen to ninety-eight) contributed.[15] Each woman was given detailed feedback on her own metagenomic results and an explanation of what they meant. But in a similar way to receiving the results of a stool test and the difficulty of interpreting the results meaningfully, the scientists involved in the project had to think very carefully about what indeed each person's results did mean (if anything), especially for women in the heterogenous CST group (Group IV) or for those with *Lactobacilli iners* (Group III).

One of the research queries that the contributors posed, and one that many women might be interested in, was whether using different sanitary products could affect the vaginal microbiome. Using pads as opposed to tampons was found to be associated with greater vaginal microbiome diversity. As with gut studies, the effects of lifestyle, age, reproductive history, contraception, diet, partners, having sex, and so forth were all looked at to see if there was an association with different microbes. Just as with the gut studies, only 8 percent of microbial variation could be explained these different parameters

The intergenerational samples obtained during the course of the ISALA study were a special set and showed that there is a measure of inheritance of the vaginal microbiome between female family members. This could fit with the likely co-evolutionary nature of this microbiome, which would require a secure method of transmission—in this case probably vertically, from mother to child, perhaps at birth, perhaps later in life between female members of the family. It is a strange but intriguing sense of connection with our ancestors, to think that some of us might be carrying the exact same strain of microbes as our great-grandmothers, and that we may have inherited specific lactobacilli from them as well as our genes.

Finally, what about sexual intercourse and its effect on the vaginal microbiome? It is well known that sperm is alkaline and alters the pH of the vagina, however temporarily, which may have an effect on the microbes present. The ISALA study was brave enough to ask its citizen scientists about their sex lives and found that those who took their swab within twenty-four hours of having sex did indeed have a more varied set of microbes present.

156 THE MICROBIOME

What about the Male Genital Microbiome?

Because of the important associated health issues to do with childbirth and post-puerperal infections, most research has gravitated toward the female genital microbiome. Research on the microbiome of the male genital tract is much sparser, and the impact on health appears to be much smaller—in a good way.

Of course, it is obvious that any sexual *infections* found in the genital tract such as syphilis, chlamydia, HIV, and so on, will have a profound impact on the patient whether male or female, on their partner and their unborn children. But what about the effect of the penis microbiome, those ordinary microbes found on the genitals of healthy men? Are these transmitted to his partner? And following sex with a female partner, is the male genital microbiome itself altered?

As is usual in microbiomes, the microbes found on each anatomical area—each habitat if we like: the foreskin, the coronal sulcus (the part just underneath the foreskin), and the urethra—are all distinct from each other and, indeed, a discussion like this would not be complete without a discussion of smegma; What is smegma? Which microbes are in smegma? And do the microbes in smegma help the host?

Smegma is the collection of cells and sebaceous material that is collected under the foreskin in boys before they are old enough to pull back the foreskin. It is normal, in fact necessary, for boys to loosen the foreskin by touching the area, and eventually most smegma is cleared away. It then continues to be produced in men in order to keep the area under the foreskin moist and lubricated. But although we can start off confidently with its definition, the amount of microbiome research on this area is so low that it's hard to take the story any further. We do know that even before the foreskin is at all retractable (for example, in young children), it is usual to find a few bacteria present in this substance, including *E. coli*, *Enterococcus avium*, and *Enterococcus faecalis* and that the microbiome of the smegma is distinct from that of the other male genital parts.

It is also known that there are more microbes found, and more variety, on the glans penis of those who are uncircumcised compared to those who are circumcised. In those who are uncircumcised, anaerobes such as *Bacteroides, Streptococci, Staphylococci, E. coli*, and *Klebsiella* are typically found in the anaerobic habitat below the foreskin. In contrast, those who are circumcised tend to have much drier skin on the glans penis, and the bacteria found there are consequently more typical of aerobic microbes found on the sebaceous or greasy skin of the body, similar to those we met in the skin chapter when talking about the microbiome of the face, such as *C. acnes, Corynebacteria*, and *Staphylococcus epidermidis*.

Is the Male Urethra Sterile?

The male urethra is the tube in the penis that drains the bladder, a rather longer structure than is found in females. When we consider if it is sterile or not, the answer is it depends on which bit. Unfortunately, the microbiome of the urethra is often conveniently assessed by taking a urine sample, in a similar way to the studies we have seen using stool as a surrogate of the microbes in the bowel. It is a strategy that can be useful, but it blurs the anatomical distinctions of the urethral microbiome. A urine sample is most accurately used when assessing the distal part of the urethra (the part closest to the opening) or when checking for STDs, but it does not distinguish between the different sections of the urethra.

In studies where urine has not been used but swabs taken of different sections of the urethra, a more accurate picture is built up. The farther away from the opening or "meatus" the urethral samples are taken, the more likely they are to be sterile. This fits both with the approach of doctors who treat the area as sterile and with what we know about the bodies innate defenses, bent toward flushing out any bacteria that have inadvertently entered, just as in the skin and the gut. Regular urination six to eight times a day of 1 to 2 liters of urine significantly reduces microbial load in the urethra in both males and females, and the acidity of the urine (pH 6.2) also discourages the presence of microbes. The presence of mucus lining the walls of the urethra, the regular shedding of urethral epithelial cells, and the antimicrobial peptides and immunoglobulin within the mucus all act together to reduce bacterial adhesion.

158 THE MICROBIOME

Metagenomic studies of the area (many based only on urine) demonstrate the usual problems of "low biomass samples" that we discussed in the neonatal chapter. Claims of a "testicular microbiome" or "urethral microbiome" have to be interpreted very carefully. Of course, these areas can become infected by microbes. It is perfectly possible to have a urinary tract infection or a testicular cellulitis. But overall, in the healthy male, the urethra is mainly sterile, with the presence of bacteria naturally becoming more common the closer we get to the opening.

Sex with a female partner does temporarily alter the male genital microbiome, particularly the microbes found in the distal part of the urethra, which can show an increase in organisms such as *Gardnerella vaginalis* and *Streptococcus agalactiae* (typical vaginal microbes).

What Is Bacterial Vaginosis?

One of the places where researchers have really got tied up in knots is with a condition known as bacterial vaginosis. This is characterized by symptoms of a watery, smelly, but non-itchy vaginal discharge, long thought to be due not so much to a vaginal infection but more an "imbalance" of the microbes, a dysbiosis. Consistent with this idea, no one microbe has ever been firmly identified as the cause of this condition. It was thought for a while that a microbe called *Gardnerella vaginalis* was the root cause, but plenty of women have bacterial vaginosis (BV) and no *Gardnerella*, and many others have *Gardnerella* but no bacterial vaginosis. Nevertheless, the standard treatment is with an antibiotic designed to treat anaerobic bacteria.

Because no pathogenic cause has been identified, it is difficult to diagnose it objectively. Two well-respected attempts include Amsel's criteria which rests on the presence of having three out of four criteria: thin, watery discharge; a vaginal pH greater than 4.5; an amine odor, and the presence of clue cells. In contrast, Nugent's criteria center on examining a vaginal smear under the microscope and detecting the presence or absence of lactobacilli, *Gardnerella*, or *Bacteroides*, ending with a score out of ten. There is a problem with both approaches. In Amsel's criteria, we know that a pH above 4.5 is normal in many women. With Nugent's criteria, there is a

The Microbiome and the Genitals   159

sort of circular reasoning; the absence of lactobacilli apparently indicating a diagnosis of bacterial vaginosis, even though this, too, is normal in some women.

Consequently, in studies using either of these criteria, BV is vastly over diagnosed, with some sources asserting that 43 percent of all women have BV and others asserting 29 percent. Other, perhaps more reasonable, studies have quoted a more likely incidence of 4 percent, although this is still a surprisingly high, implying that one in twenty women walking past us in the street is suffering from a watery, smelly discharge—an assertion that many family doctors seeing women all the time would be unlikely to agree with.[16]

According to these criteria, many young women, up to 40 percent in some ethnic groups, have smears characteristic of BV even though they have never had sex, perhaps implying it is something they have always had or perhaps have even inherited from their own mothers or own communities. It may be that what researchers have really been doing here is identifying women with the more variable, anaerobic bacteria analogous to CST Group IV.[17][18]

Ploughing on with their diagnoses of BV, researchers have long wondered if this condition might be associated with premature birth, even though prematurity is well known to be multifactorial. Large trials, including one recently on more than 6,000 pregnant women, have found that diagnosing and treating BV does not significantly change the number of premature babies born.[19]

Considering this confusion about BV and the differing but normal CST groups, should we be using the term "dysbiosis"? Or should the concept of dysbiosis be abandoned as too vague, too nonspecific and used to mean too many things? In theory, the word "dysbiosis" means "a shift away from the healthy ratios of species in the microbiota that could lead to a disrupted ecosystem that could harm the host," not an unreasonable idea and intellectually interesting. But examples of this kind of dysbiosis are surprisingly few and far between, and the term is usually used to describe the kind of altered microbiomes we see in many medical conditions.

Because the concept has become so vague, some scientists are suggesting that we drop it altogether. It is no longer news that ill people end up with

160 THE MICROBIOME

a different microbiome compared to healthy people. For the term dysbiosis to be useful, we need to be able to show that changes in the microbiome can cause disease or, at the very least, predict disease.

In the case of women with symptoms of bacterial vaginosis, an antibiotic is still the first line treatment. However, in those with recurrent BV in whom antibiotics have not worked, until a proven vaginal probiotic is available, the best we can advise women is that we get our healthy vaginal microbiomes from our female relatives and friends, from living together, and from close contact and hugs.

Perhaps, from a medical point of view, we are best off sticking to the well-known messages of safe sex and contraception, condoms, and regular sexual health checks that our kind and responsible high school teachers taught us. For doctors, to continue to follow key WHO advice on safe childbirth management, handwashing, avoiding vaginal examinations, and adhering to "standard infection prevention and control" measures—rather than adding anything extra related to what we have found out about the male and female genital microbiomes. And should we ever be unlucky enough to contract a serious post-puerperal infection or an STD, we know that although it's against all the advice on how to preserve our microbiomes, we are lucky enough to have access to effective antibiotics that might possibly save our lives.

8

PROBIOTICS AND THE MICROBIOME INDUSTRY

Many of us may be particularly interested in probiotics. In fact, it may be the thing people are most curious about in a book on the microbiome—not just how our microbiomes impact on our gut, our skin, our babies, or our sex lives, but how we do something about it. Some of us may even be taking probiotics right now and perhaps wondering whether they actually help or not.

What Are Probiotics?

Most of us know what probiotics are. They are "friendly bacteria" in the form of tablets, powders, or drinks –supplements with live bacteria in them that are meant to top up our gut bacteria and improve our health. They are thought by many of us to be natural, beneficial, and healthy and are extremely popular dietary supplements. Slogans like "Helps support your digestive health" help us to work out what probiotics are for and what they do. When we see these well-packaged products in prime positions on our supermarket shelves, it encourages us to think that these are quality products, worth paying for.

The official World Health Organization (WHO) definition of a probiotic is "live microorganisms that, when administered in adequate amounts, confer a health benefit on the host." This is a key definition and is widely quoted. It appears everywhere: from the publications (admittedly with

162 THE MICROBIOME

vested interests) of the International Scientific Association for Probiotics and Prebiotics, to newspaper articles, patient leaflets, and the regulatory bodies of every country.

The probiotic market is buoyant and has increased more than threefold in the past two decades, with over 4.5 percent of US adults and children regularly taking them. Their use is especially prevalent among older people and those with higher educational levels, higher incomes, and better diets.[1]

As well as probiotics, there are many other products marketed by the microbiome industry. Prebiotics are one. These are substances designed to pass undigested through our digestive tracts to provide nutrients for our gut microbes. Depending on which we take, these "selectively encourage the growth of certain beneficial species," and are intended to confer a health benefit as a result.[2] Synbiotics are another. These are a combination of probiotics and prebiotics meant to act "synergistically," hence their name.[3] The idea that certain foods are indigestible to us but fermentable by microbes is a key aspect of the microbiome, as we saw in the gut chapter, and appears to be a great concept for a microbiome health product. We might expect fiber to be a good example and breast milk another. However, confusingly, neither fiber nor breast milk strictly count as prebiotics because these foods promote *groups* of microbes rather than just one. This suggests that the definition is perhaps too narrow to be useful, especially as we are well aware that the gut microbiome is all about groups or varieties of microbes.[4]

Postbiotics are another example of a microbiome product, but one from which the microbes have been filtered out, killed, or inactivated, leaving behind the (presumed) bioactive substances. While this is an intriguing and potent idea, it clearly overlaps with other well-established scientific concepts and products such as antibiotics and certain vaccines, and the exact definition of a postbiotic is still hotly debated.[5]

Fermented foods too are a well-known and very popular category of microbiome-enhancing health foods right now. These include foods and drinks *purposely* fermented by microbes (not just gone moldy) either to preserve the food, to improve its flavor, its nutritional content, or to make it alcoholic. Examples include foods and drinks that end up with no microbes in them at all, such as wine, bread, and coffee, as well as foods that have a great number of microbes in them, such as salami, cheese, yogurt, sour cream, kefir, kimchi, sauerkraut, miso, soy sauce, and many other examples found all over the world. The microbes involved in fermented foods don't have to be bacteria; they can be yeasts or even a combination of yeasts and bacteria, as is the case for cider vinegar. Nor do fermented foods have to be literally fermented: there are various chemical pathways that can enzymatically convert food.

The fermented food industry (and the probiotic industry) insists that fermented foods are distinct from probiotics, as probiotics necessarily have to have a "health benefit" and specify the strains and doses of the microbes within them to be classified as such, whereas fermented foods do not. Having said that, many fermented foods do mention which live bacteria are present, immediately blurring the boundary between the two products.

Although we love fermented foods and drinks (they honestly account for approximately one-third of the human diet)—it is clear that they are not automatically healthy. This is obvious when we consider the alcohol we consume in wine and beer, or the salt contained in miso and soy sauce. Many fermented products contain lots of dead microbes (similar in concept to postbiotics), products with live microbes do sometimes survive to reach the colon, as we discussed in the gut chapter, but don't usually maintain a long-term presence.

What Other Products Does the Microbiome Industry Support?

As well as the various therapeutic and dietary formulations already mentioned, the microbiome industry also encompasses an extensive range of other products, which support scientists in producing the exponentially increasing volume of microbiome research. This is evident from a quick glance at the sponsors supporting microbiome conferences, which themselves represent a lucrative segment of the microbiome industry. These various microbiome industry offshoots offer diverse and sometimes unexpected services, from a full microbiome analysis to DNA extraction kits for scientists to do the analysis themselves.

164 THE MICROBIOME

Companies providing products for collecting microbiome samples in the field, DNA extraction reagents for lab work, synthetic mucus for in vitro studies, and germ-free mice for in vivo testing all support and are part of the microbiome industry. Additionally, there are companies offering to process samples using metagenomics or other techniques and others specializing in bioinformatic analyses alone, with huge libraries of microbial DNA sequences *not* freely available online. There is also the communication industry, including companies such as MicrobiomePost, Teknoscienze, and Microbiomejournal, which exist to communicate the massive output of microbiome research. It is clear that the microbiome industry is experiencing rapid growth driven by both advancements in sequencing technologies and exponentially increasing volumes of research. Although valued at approximately $800 million at the present time, the global microbiome market size is projected to reach over $3,000 million by 2031.

Where Did the Idea of Manipulating Our Gut Microbes Originate?

The idea of manipulating our gut microbes first started with an important and influential Russian zoologist Elie Metchnikoff (1845–1916). He was awarded the Nobel Prize for his work on immunity in 1908 and later became subdirector of the Pasteur Institute. He is often given the moniker "father of probiotics," as he was the first to promote the eating of yogurt with live cultures to promote good health and longevity.

But if you think his promotion of yogurt way back in 1903 shows that he thought the human gut microbiome needed to be "nourished," "revitalized" or "topped up," you couldn't be more wrong. In fact, he thought the complete opposite.

Far from being the "father of probiotics" Metchnikoff thought that bacteria in the large colon were pointless—even dangerous. He subscribed to the theory current at the time that colonic bacteria caused "autointoxication"; that bacterial waste products rotting away in the gut leached into the human circulatory system, causing headaches, depression, mental sluggishness, and irritability. This fits closely with the theories connecting the gut and the mind current in the late 19th century, that we discussed in the gut-brain chapter.[6] In his view, the microbes that multiplied unceasingly within our guts caused untold harm to our bodies, literally shortening our lives. "The accumulation of waste matter retained in the large intestine for considerable periods becomes a nidus for microbes which produce fermentation and putrefaction." His whole goal was to reduce the number of bacteria in the colon.

He considers a number of different ways to achieve this and describes them in his book *The Prolongation of Life, Optimistic Studies*. He starts with dietary measures—including a suggestion to eat only cooked food or, alternatively, only sterilized food—but finds that this "by no means causes the disappearance of the intestinal flora already existing." He also considers the idea of chewing food more thoroughly to enable it to be more fully absorbed in the small intestine, which would leave less undigested matter for microbes to use.[7]

Direct use of antiseptics within the gut is another approach that he discusses in detail, and he quotes various colleagues of his who self-experiment using this technique. However, neither purgative options such as calomel nor disinfectant chemicals like beta-naphthol (used in the dyeing industry and thought to be "moderately toxic"), naphthalene (used in mothballs and now known to be carcinogenic), or camphor were effective. In fact, following the use of these agents, intestinal microbes *"even increased in numbers."*

Although we may be turning our noses up right now at this approach, the concept of decontaminating the large bowel is still in use today in some intensive care units, both in America and Europe. Known as "selective decontamination of the digestive tract" (SDD), this practice involves the use of intravenous antibiotics and six hourly administrations of an oral antibiotic paste and gastric suspensions. It is given to intensive care patients with the intention to prevent infections, although the latest trials do not show significantly reduced mortality.[8]

It is when Metchnikoff discusses the worldwide use of fermented foods, commenting on the good health of those eating these traditional foods, that he really latches onto something: "On this diet they enjoy excellent health, display great vigour and reach advanced ages."

166 THE MICROBIOME

"M. Grigoroff, a Bulgarian student at Geneva, has been surprised by the number of centenarians to be found in Bulgaria, a region in which yahourth, a soured milk, is the stable food. Some of the centenarians, described by M. Chemin in his memoir, lived chiefly on a milk diet. Marie Priou, for example, who died in the Haute-Garonne in 1838 at the age of 158 years, had lived for the last ten years of her life entirely on cheese and goat's milk. Ambroise Jantet, a labourer of Verdun, who died in 1751 at the age of 111 years, "ate nothing but unleavened bread and drank nothing but skimmed milk." Nicole Marc, who died aged 110 years, at the chateau of Colemberg (Pas-de-Calais), a hunch-back and cripple, "lived only on bread and milk-food"."

Metchnikoff was well aware that the lactic acid produced by lactic acid bacilli used to make fermented milk prevented other bacteria from growing, but he takes the idea much further: "As lactic fermentation serves so well to arrest putrefaction in general, why should it not be used for the same purpose within the digestive tube?"

He obtained a specimen of the Bulgarian "yahourth" from the aforementioned Monsieur Grigoroff, isolated the most active lactic bacillus that he could find, and named it *Bulgarian bacillus*. Now known as *Lactobacillus delbrueckii* subspecies *Bulgaricus*, it is still widely used today.

He then explained to thousands of people in sell-out talks that taking his lactobacillus in yogurt would allow them to live longer, healthier lives. He himself consumed yogurt every day after that, dying at the age of 71 from heart failure. Although eating yogurt did not noticeably prolong his own life, his beliefs about yogurt and live cultures are incredibly influential. Even today, we can't escape from the feeling that yogurt *is* a healthy food, even though we know logically that it depends on how much we eat and who we are (for example, it wouldn't be especially healthy for a patient with a milk protein intolerance).

Some people will wonder why he encouraged the consumption of billions of yogurt microbes when he was so against intestinal microbes. But as he explained, "There are many useful microbes, amongst which the lactic bacilli have an honourable place."

We have talked in detail about Metchnikoff, not because he is necessarily right about reducing the colonic microbial load or even about the healthful effects of probiotics and fermented foods, but because he seems to have invented the entire microbiome industry.

As well as producing the first-ever probiotic (*Bulgarian bacillus*), he seems to have invented the whole idea of altering gut microbes to improve health. He introduced the idea of chemical treatments to decontaminate the gut which, as we have seen, are still used today. He suggested dietary manipulation to alter the gut microbiome, introducing the concept of *pre*biotics. He also promoted the use of fermented foods as healthy, a belief that remains widespread, and was the first to selectively isolate a strain of lactobacillus for certain qualities, now a standard procedure in probiotic selection. Finally, although not discussed here, he describes in his book experiments in which solutions of killed *Bulgarian bacillus* are administered to mice and shown to improve their health, thereby inventing the concept of *post*biotics as well.

What Would Make an Effective Probiotic?

Obviously, the world of probiotics has evolved somewhat since Metchnikoff selected his *Lactobacillus* strain, but as we can see, he set the standard. He considered the health benefit he was looking for and selected the microbe that would provide it.

But there are other key theoretical attributes that a modern probiotic manufacturer might also wish to select for. As well as needing a specific microbe that can reach the customer alive (Metchnikoff achieved this) a probiotic microbe ideally should also survive to reach the gut or "target organ," stay in the gut and proliferate, interact with the host, and confer a health benefit.

To gain a toehold in the gut and make a home for themselves, bacteria are said to stick themselves to the epithelial cells lining the intestinal tract, using tiny bacterial structures such as fimbriae (little threads) that protrude from the cell walls. This is a quality known as "mucosal adherence" and the idea of being able to remain in the gut and then to multiply and thrive is known as "engrafting." It would seem likely that a probiotic would have to engraft to significantly interact with a host. However, some scientists do argue that a probiotic can cause a health benefit without engrafting, simply by being present temporarily.

Once a start-up probiotics company has identified a strain that has achieved all of these goals, then from point of view of commercialization, the product has to be stable, reproducible, palatable, and have an acceptable shelf life.

A new probiotic strain will need to be scaled up with the help of a fermentation company, some of which have long histories, having been producing microbes for the dairy industry since the 19th century. They are used to implementing stringent cleanliness routines and will tweak the growing conditions to get the microbes proliferating at maximum capabilities in huge steel vats. The mixture is then freeze-dried into solid cakes and milled into powder, ready to be formed into tablets.[9] At every stage, the product is checked for culture yields per milliliter, and although only about 20 percent of microbes survive from vat to tablet (the milling is especially destructive), this still typically yields a massive 100 trillion microbes per gram of product.

What Are Some Examples of Well-Known Probiotic Microbes?

There is a profusion of probiotics available, with hundreds available globally and more than ninety just in the United States. They are used for a wide range of gastrointestinal conditions, including ulcerative colitis, Crohn's disease, irritable bowel syndrome, constipation, acute diarrhea, traveler's diarrhea, antibiotic-associated diarrhea, and various other non-gut-related conditions such as eczema, asthma, autism, urinary tract infections, rheumatoid arthritis, diabetes, and many others. They are some specifically marketed for certain patient groups: the elderly, children, patients in intensive care units and premature babies. And as well as all of this, probiotics are sometimes marketed for "healthy people" to make them . . . more healthy. Which, aside from that fact that no one can yet define the word "healthy," is a very interesting claim indeed.

As we have already seen, *Lactobacillus delbrueckii* subspecies *Bulgaricus* was the first-ever probiotic made, and it is also one of a select group of microbes that still dominate the market. As well as our *Bulgaricus*, this group includes Henri Tissier's *Bifidobacteria*, isolated in France and first used as a therapy for children by him in 1906; Alfred Nissle's *E. coli* strain, isolated in Germany in 1917 from a soldier who appeared to be resistant to a Shigella outbreak; Minoru Shirota's *Lactobacillus casei* Shirota strain, isolated in Japan in 1930 and selected for its ability to survive the digestive tract—still marketed today as Yakult; and finally, *Saccharomyces boulardii*, a yeast isolated by Henri Boulard in 1923 from the skin of fruit after he noticed the Vietnamese chewing lychee peel to control the symptoms of cholera.[10]

There are a few others that have been isolated more recently: *Lactobacillus rhamnosus* GG, isolated by Gorbach and Goldin in America from human feces in 1983 and named after themselves; *Lactobacillus reuteri*, isolated from breast milk in Peru in 1990; and *Lactobacillus helveticus*, identified in an acidophilus milk starter, also in 1990.

When we consider the number of microbes in the world, or even just within our guts, one might imagine there would be thousands of probiotic microbes on the market. Yet, oddly, most probiotics feature just one or a group of this limited handful of species. For example, a typical product might include a consortium of six strains: *Lactobacillus rhamnosus Consi-04, Lactobacillus acidophilus/helveticus Consi-46, Bifidobacterium longum Consi-541, Bifidobacterium breve Consi-30, Bifidobacterium bifidum Consi-14*, and *Lactococcus lactis Consi-1032*. Here we see three strains of bifidobacterium, a microbe that naturally accounts for about 3 percent of our gut microbes anyway, and three lactic acid bacilli, each frequently used in the dairy industry—so microbes that we might already be consuming anyway.

Are Probiotics Regulated?

The manufacturing and labeling of probiotics *is* regulated, but perhaps in a somewhat relaxed and lenient manner. Products must be labeled with the names of each microorganism and the total number of colony-forming units (CFU) per dose (not including any inactive, dead, or nonviable organisms)

170 THE MICROBIOME

listed in order of weight. We can infer from the theoretical probiotic product material listed above, for example, that *Lactobacillus rhamnosus* would account for the largest number of microbes present, while *Lactococcus lactis* would account for the least.[11]

The strangely limited list of microbes used in probiotics that we have outlined above can be somewhat explained by industry guidelines. By rule, probiotics can only contain microbes that are "generally recognized as safe" (GRAS), implying that there is "scientific agreement about a substance's safety based on appropriate testing or common use in food before 1958." A product with GRAS status can then be marketed with no further safety testing.

Once identified as GRAS, probiotics are then typically labeled with a "qualified health claim," which usually takes the form of a "structure/function" claim. This can be quite nonspecific for example, "promotes digestion". Along with a structure/function claim, the packaging material must also include a disclaimer that the claim "has not been evaluated by the Food and Drug Administration (FDA)" and that the product is "not intended to diagnose, treat, cure, or prevent disease." It's interesting to note that qualified health claims are permissible even if they are only "potentially misleading." Some have said that this has allowed the probiotics industry to have experienced almost exponential growth driven by creative marketing.[12]

Probiotic manufacturers have in the past been taken to court, however, for using misleading advertising and have had to retract several claims, including "scientifically proven to help support your kid's defenses," "helps to maintain [contributes to] the intestinal defense function," "improves gastrointestinal comfort," and "helps to strengthen the body's natural defenses". They are now perhaps more cautious in their claims of health benefits.[13] But even with just these indefinite and non-specific claims, the probiotic industry has managed to convey some very strong messages: that probiotics are good for us, that they help our immune system, and that they improve gut symptoms of all sorts. Consumers are apparently as likely to use probiotics for diarrhea as they are for constipation.[14]

Conversely, some of the claims on probiotic packaging are surprisingly restrained and probably completely true: "scientifically proven to reach the gut alive," "includes strains extensively studied for 20 years," and even (frankly undermining their own utility) "*Lactobacillus, Bifidobacterium*, and *Lactococcus* naturally occur in the digestive tract." Here, there are no health claims to be seen at all—not even a suggestion that probiotics are for healthy people.

It is not surprising that probiotics stick to their GRAS status and their limited structure/function claims because as well as being expensive, a trial process would require that the product be completely taken off the market as an "unapproved drug" until the health claim had been settled. As the market is flourishing so well using GRAS status and without specific health claims, there is no incentive for suppliers to conduct trials at all.

But just because the probiotic industry has chosen not to jump through trial hoops does not automatically mean that probiotics do not work, nor does it mean that probiotics have not been tested. Countless studies on probiotics have been carried out by other stakeholders. There have been many claims made about the clinical efficacy of probiotics: that they improve gastric ulcer healing, that they reduce inflammation, that they treat diarrhea (or constipation), and many others.

Following positive results for probiotics in some trials, researchers have then tried to explain how probiotics work, detailing their effect on the immune system, on the stress axis, on suppressing pathogens, on the balance of the microbiome, on how they restore essential gut microbes, and how they improve the barrier function of gut epithelial cells.[15]

What Does the Research on Probiotics Show?

The probiotic studies that we do have, have mostly been of the medical kind, the "does it work or not?" sort—not an unreasonable approach in the first instance. These typically measure symptom rates, such as the number of diarrhea stools per day, and compare rates in a treated group to an untreated group. Ideally, this kind of trial is conducted as a "double-blind trial," where neither healthcare staff nor patients know if they have been given the active treatment or the placebo. Studies like this have been conducted on probiotics for any number of conditions.

Given the amount of research, it is disappointing that the evidence for probiotics is weak, to say the least. Many early studies on probiotics (and, in fact, recent ones too) are small, based on fewer than 30–40 patients, making the results less likely to be reliable. Combining studies to get the patient numbers and statistical strength of a big trial is one way around this problem. For example, the well-respected Cochrane group published a meta-analysis of probiotics to prevent antibiotic-associated diarrhea (AAD), which combined thirty-three studies and reached a total of 6,352 participants. But there are problems with this approach. Meta-analyses are famously flawed by publication bias, and for any study showing an effect, there are a notable number of others that have been registered but never published because of boring negative results, undermining the conclusion of the analysis. As well, probiotic meta-analyses have the unique problem, in that trials using different probiotic *microbes* are often lumped together. If each microbe genuinely has a different effect, this makes a nonsense of the conclusions (see note 15).

The gastrointestinal specialties have taken a particular interest in the probiotic studies and meta-analyses that we do have. It is they who need to be able to advise their patients about when to use probiotics, and it is they who have published guidelines on their use. Their guideline development is typically thorough, with a full panel of specialists, public consultations, and a carefully curated literature search.

It is exciting to see an aspect of the microbiome world finally entering into both the British and American guidelines, but the news is not good for probiotics. Consider the following quotes from the American Gastroenterological Association (AGA) 2020 guidelines:

For ulcerative colitis: "recommends the use of probiotics only in the context of a clinical trial. No recommendation; knowledge gap."

For Crohn's disease: "recommends the use of probiotics only in the context of a clinical trial. No recommendation; knowledge gap."

For irritable bowel, infectious diarrhea, and all the other potential gastrointestinal indications, the same. For acute gastroenteritis: "we suggest against the use of probiotics" —not exactly a ringing endorsement.

In fact, the American guidelines do not advise probiotics for anything except, possibly, maybe antibiotic-associated diarrhea in children, but with a warning tacked into the middle: "conditional recommendation, low quality of evidence."[16]

Do Probiotics Work for Antibiotic Associated Diarrhea?

Antibiotic-associated diarrhea is one of the very few concrete examples we have of a proven dysbiosis where probiotics might reasonably be expected to help. Antibiotics really do alter the balance of microbes in our gut, and metagenomic studies of patients clearly document a perturbation of the gut bacteria, sometimes even with the loss of certain species if subjected to several courses. Overall, the research shows that gut microbes do go more or less back to normal within a week in most people after a course of antibiotics, although in some it can take up to two months.[17]

The great majority of us don't get any gut symptoms or diarrhea at all when we take antibiotics. However, about one in ten children (more in the younger ones) do experience antibiotic-associated diarrhea, defined as three soft stools for at least forty-eight hours, typically starting two to five days after a course of antibiotics has been initiated.[18] Antibiotic-associated diarrhea is thought to occur because the reduction in the usual bacteria that ferment our indigestible fiber leads to more fiber remaining in the gut, causing looser stools (see note 18).

Both the American and British guidelines cite the Cochrane meta-analysis mentioned above, which advises that probiotics apparently have a small positive effect. For every ten children on antibiotics who are given probiotics, one child might be helped, and the amount of diarrhea reduced by one day. They recommend either *Lactobacillus rhamnosus* or *Saccharomyces boulardii* probiotics at a dosage of 5–40 billion CFU per day.[19]

One other guideline recommends probiotics: a British guideline for irritable bowel syndrome, which suggests "a trial of probiotics for up to 12 weeks," discontinued if there is no improvement.[20]

Just to be clear here, the Cochrane advice suggests that *either* a bacteria *or* a yeast is equally effective, and the dose they recommend ranges tenfold—recommendations that could be described as being somewhat casual. Perhaps they are made on the basis that probiotics can't do any harm and may even do some good, so we might as well try them. But should we be so casual? Probiotic capsules include massive numbers of microbes, sometimes over 100 billion microbes in a single dose—more than we might come across naturally in a month. Surely, the safety of probiotics is something we should be taking seriously.

Are Probiotics Safe?

As we have already seen, probiotics *are* widely regarded as safe and are sold based on their "generally recognized as safe" status. These are typically benign microbes, and many have been used in fermented foods for generations. They do not spore, they are non-motile, and they mostly do not exhibit any of the characteristics of pathogens: no toxins, no flagella.[21] In any case, our innate immune system is highly effective. Most microbes—including probiotic ones—don't make it past the acid in our stomach.

However, probiotics are still microbes, and 100 billion is not the level of microbes that our body's immune system is used to handling. Even the relatively high numbers of microbes found in fermented foods do not reach these kinds of levels (usually more at the million microbes per portion kind of level). If they get in the wrong part of our body, even "benign" microbes can cause an infection.

But in spite of the fact that we are administering live microbes, safety issues and side effects associated with probiotics are not taken seriously. Nearly a third of probiotic trials don't bother mentioning data related to harms, and 80 percent give no data at all on serious adverse events.[22,23]

Serious adverse events have occurred, but without trials properly documenting them and bringing probiotic safety issues to people's attention, prescriptions for probiotics have continued to rise. There has been a documented three-fold increase in probiotics prescribed by doctors in US hospitals over recent decades, often particularly administered to patients who have had antibiotics or those who are seriously ill.[24]

Patients with severe acute pancreatitis are a good example of individuals who are seriously ill. These patients are at risk of infectious complications from small bowel bacterial overgrowth and mucosal barrier failure, and these two failures of the immune system can lead to the translocation of intestinal bacteria into the bloodstream, causing septicemia. Despite these known facts, 298 patients with severe pancreatitis were enrolled in a probiotic trial and given a multi-species probiotic containing 10 billion microbes "to prevent infectious complications." In this study, twenty-four patients (16 percent) in the probiotics group died, compared to nine (6 percent) in the placebo group; eight of those in the probiotics group died from bowel ischemia (none died from this in the placebo group).[25]

In another probiotic trial, six intensive care patients dosed with *Lactobacillus rhamnosus* GG (known to translocate from the bowel to the bloodstream more often than other probiotics) ended up with life-threatening bacteremia. All six patients were confirmed by whole genome sequencing to be infected with the exact same strain they had been dosed with.[26]

Reports of proven probiotic sepsis in premature babies are also not uncommon. Indeed, given how awkward it would be for a clinician to report a probiotic sepsis, especially if fatal, cases are probably underreported.[27] However, probiotics continue to be frequently used in premature babies in a desperate attempt to manage the life-threatening condition necrotizing enterocolitis and have been found to spread unintentionally, detected in the stool of untreated premature babies in the same unit, probably transferred on the hands of healthcare staff.[28]

Whole genome sequencing has clearly demonstrated that these infections are caused by probiotics, proving that probiotics cannot ever be considered completely harmless. These are live microbial agents given at

176 THE MICROBIOME

high levels, which can cause life-threatening infections if they get into the wrong place. This information is at last piercing through the wall of advertising to reach patient information leaflets, (even if it has not yet reached the ears of their doctors). The leaflets pragmatically conclude that, although probiotics are safe in the vast majority, "there is a small risk of adverse effects, such as sepsis. It is therefore recommended that use of these agents be avoided in those who are immunocompromised, severely debilitated, critically ill or postoperative, as this population is most at risk."[29]

What Do Metagenomic Techniques Have to Say about Probiotics?

It has to be admitted that there are some strange contradictions inherent in our use of and enthusiasm for probiotics, given what we now know about the microbiome. Conventional probiotics are facultative anaerobes, but most of the bacteria in our gut are anaerobic. We love taking probiotics, but probiotics for the most part consist of microbes that we already have. A wide variety of species is widely agreed to indicate a healthy gut, but probiotic formulations often consist of just one. Probiotics are live microbes, but we act as if they cannot cause infections.

We know why Metchnikoff wanted to give lactobacilli. He thought a large growth of lactic acid producing bacilli would reduce the numbers of other bacteria in the colon and prevent patients from suffering from "autotoxaemia." But we are still promoting the consumption of lactobacilli today, even though we no longer believe in autotoxaemia, but the exact opposite: that a varied, thriving community of bacteria in the colon is healthy.

But the microbiome research community is keen to shed some light on what is really happening in our guts when we take a dose of probiotics. Metagenomic techniques can look in huge detail at the gut microbial community and are well placed to improve our understanding of this topic, unpick these contradictions, and show if probiotics engraft or not.

Suez et al., working in Tel Aviv, Israel, have really got to the bottom of this debate with their thorough and meticulous approach. By using colonoscopies and taking mucosal biopsies throughout the gastrointestinal tract in fifteen healthy subjects, both before and after a course of probiotics, the team showed that although probiotics are found in the stool (temporarily) after a dose, they are not found in the mucosal microarchitecture. This suggests that in most healthy people probiotics don't usually engraft. It appears that probiotic microbes are simply not finding a foothold in an established and stable gut microbiome.

When they repeated the study on subjects dosed with antibiotics first to simulate antibiotic-associated dysbiosis, they found that the probiotics had a higher chance of engrafting. Although most people were still "non-responders," "responders" did end up with the probiotic microbe living on in their gut long-term, causing a definite change to their gut microbiome. In those in whom the probiotic had not engrafted, there was no change to the balance of their usual gut microbiome, thus ending the debate on whether a probiotic has to engraft to have an effect. It does.[30]

However, in those patients where the probiotic had engrafted, the probiotic did no good. It got in the way, delaying the return of their usual microbiomes and actually causing a demonstrable reduction in the numbers and species of other bacteria within the colon. Amazingly, it appears that Metchnikoff's theory has been proven correct: Lactobacilli really do reduce the numbers of colonic bacteria; it's just that we no longer think this is desirable.[31]

It's not just metagenomic studies that have finally given us some clear answers. A recently conducted large, randomized, quadruple-blind, placebo-controlled trial involving 350 pediatric patients taking a 10-billion-multispecies probiotic to prevent antibiotic-associated diarrhea (exactly as recommended by the Cochrane review) found no effect whatsoever on the rates of diarrhea.[32]

And an even bigger trial on 2,940 adult patients dosed with a 6-billion-multistrain probiotic to prevent antibiotic-associated diarrhea again found no effect.[33]

If it's true that probiotics have little or no effect on the healthy gut and a negative or even detrimental effect in those with antibiotic-associated diarrhea, it's embarrassing to contemplate all the work done on explaining how probiotics "work." Theories explaining how probiotics modulate the

178 THE MICROBIOME

immune system and alter the stress axis are apparently made to appear ludicrous.

But something else *does* work for returning the gut to normal after a course of antibiotics, a different treatment entirely: fecal microbiota transplants (FMTs). Suez's team demonstrated that oral treatment with an autologous fecal microbiota transplant following a course of antibiotics returned the gut microbiota completely back to normal within two days.[34]

What Is a Faecal Microbiota Transplant?

An FMT is basically a stool transplant. It is putting someone else's stool, a donor stool, into the colon of a patient. If using an autologous stool transplant, as in Suez's study, the patient's own stool (obtained before the course of antibiotics or before they were ill) is used.

If you are reading this and wrinkling up your nose and wondering about the practicalities of a stool transplant, that's perfectly understandable; it is a bit gross. We have spent generations avoiding touching, seeing, or even smelling stool if we can help it (with the help of flush toilets). But many animals don't feel the same way. Some are obliged to eat their stool as part of their usual nutrition (so don't clean your guinea pig's cages out too often because these animals are one of them). Other animals also find feces deeply interesting. You may have previously found this out if you have a dog that has deliberately eaten some poop and then come indoors and tried to lick your face. Even chimpanzees are known to pass a nice log and then start eating it (you may be feeling slightly sick reading this).

But stool transplants really do work for certain conditions, sometimes effecting a cure within hours. As well as working for antibiotic-associated diarrhea, they are particularly effective for *Clostridium difficile* infections.

What Is a Clostridium difficile Infection?

A *Clostridium difficile* infection is a bacterial infection of the large colon, causing severe bloody and sometimes life-threatening diarrhea, often triggered by a course of oral antibiotics. It is believed to be caused by an imbalance of the colonic bacteria that, decimated by the antibiotics, allows an overgrowth of *Clostridium difficile* bacterium to cause an infection. Although this bacterium is usually a normal part of our gut microbiome, it can take over and cause a very serious illness, in some patients progressing to a life-threatening condition known as pseudomembranous colitis. *C. diff* infections are a persistent infection control issue in hospitals, and it can spread rapidly between patients.

Most strains of *Clostridium difficile* are not pathogenic, though, and various strains of this bacterium are present in about 3 percent of healthy adults and 66 percent of infants. First described by Hall and O'Toole in 1935 (whom we met in the newborn chapter), it was obtained from the stool of healthy infants; an anaerobic, sporing bacteria, very difficult to grow, hence its original name: *Bacillus difficile*.[35]

As antibiotics began to be used more and more over the next two decades, the negative consequences of their use began to be felt, and the incidence of *C. diff* infections and pseudomembranous colitis began to increase. Meanwhile, in Colorado in 1958, the first documented use of a fecal transplant for pseudomembranous colitis was reported.

A surgeon named B. Eiseman appears to have made this idea up, completely out of his own head, admitting the fact in interviews years later. "This therapy is based upon the fact that [bacterial] overgrowth occurs when other organisms disappear and that re-introduction of the bacteria, viruses and bacteriophage normally found in the colon might re-establish the balance of nature with subsidence of . . . the distressing symptoms caused thereby." Eiseman wrote up six patients who had been completely moribund with pseudomembranous colitis and whom he had treated with stool transplants. It worked, literally within hours, bringing these patients back from the brink of death.[36]

Although incredibly effective and used by Eiseman throughout his career, the idea of fecal transplants has been slow to take off, moving only slowly toward acceptability, standard therapy, and finally a commercial product. This has recently been approved for medical use and is at last entering standard guidelines for the treatment of recurrent *Clostridium difficile* infections.

180 THE MICROBIOME

These guidelines advise that stool for administration should be centrifuged, filtered, frozen, and stored in stool banks. When used, it must be given within hours of defrosting and administered as a liquid per rectum (not via a naso-gastro tube due to the risk of aspiration pneumonia). Alternatively, freeze-dried gastric-protected tablets can be used, as Suez used in his antibiotic-associated diarrhea study.[37,38]

But although FMTs are now established as an effective therapy, they are rarely used. The National Registry for FMTs, reflecting real-world practice, has recorded only 259 usages over two years (although with a 90 percent cure rate), and first-line treatment is still intravenous vancomycin antibiotic. But actually neither FMTs nor antibiotics should be first for a *C. diff* outbreak. The first approach should be prevention.[39]

The incidence of *C. diff* infection is reduced by using broad-spectrum antibiotics only when absolutely necessary. When suspected, early screening is essential and barrier nursing mandatory. It is public health measures that keep the rates of this serious infection down, not FMTs.

Although not first-line treatment for either *C. diff* infections or antibiotic-associated diarrhea, FMTs really do work. The excitement generated by the amazing success rates of this procedure has encouraged clinicians to try FMTs for many other conditions, from inflammatory bowel disease to irritable bowel syndrome. Unfortunately, the same sort of success has not been demonstrated for these or indeed any other indications, leading to frustrations among patients who just want to give the process a try. In the face of resistance from their medical practitioners, some people have even turned to doing it themselves, leading to the phenomenon of do-it-yourself (DIY) FMTs.

What Are DIY Faecal Microbiota Transplants?

Just to be clear, DIY FMTs are not recommended here. The evidence and the guidelines, both American and European, do not recommend FMT for anything except recurrent *C. diff* infections. In addition, there are many safety issues and uncertainties remaining with regard to FMT, including how to screen donors, what tests to do on donated stools, and the many long-term unknowns associated with this procedure.

But these concerns haven't stopped the phenomenon of DIY FMTs taking off following explicit instructions on the internet regarding turkey basters.[40] A questionnaire filled out by a self-selected group of people visiting popular fecal transplant internet sites found that, instead of the stool donor remaining anonymous as is usual, 92 percent totally knew their donors. And although people are self-treating for many expected conditions, they are also using FMTs for less-orthodox indications, including obesity, autoimmune disorders, and neuropsychiatric conditions such as depression and autism. Over 40 percent had repeated the procedure more than ten times, with the great majority (82 percent) reporting a marked improvement in their symptoms.

Choosing to do an FMT on oneself is one thing and is eye-opening enough, but the fact that 12 percent of this group had performed an FMT on their children makes this unregulated practice significantly more concerning.

Are Any Other Microbiome Therapies in the Pipeline?

There is one other condition for which FMTs have recently been found effective: certain cancer patients receiving immune-modulating chemotherapy. Phase I trials have already proven that FMTs are safe in these patients, and early indications suggest that they genuinely improve the response rate to checkpoint inhibitor chemotherapy, though further trials will be needed to prove their effectiveness.[41]

There have also been transplants of other parts of our microbiome. Skin microbiome transplants have been tried for people with intractable body odor, where skin bacteria from a healthy donor's axilla have been transplanted to recipients with good results. There have also been vaginal microbiota transplants successfully used to treat intractable bacterial vaginosis and, in one proof-of-concept case, as a treatment for infertility.[42,43]

There is also research indicating that just taking fiber can help modulate the microbiome in patients with cancer. Patients undergoing radiotherapy respond very well to regular doses of fiber, which appears to protect the gut epithelial cells from radiation, thereby mitigating side effects.[44]

182 THE MICROBIOME

Live biotherapeutic products (LBPs) are another exciting development. Sometimes also known as novel probiotics, these are similar to conventional probiotics in that they contain live microbes, but different because they are not long known to the food industry or recognized as safe. They include newly selected microbes of quite different species compared to classic probiotics. Because they are not "generally recognized as safe," LBPs have had to follow a completely different regulatory path, one more similar to that used for novel drug development. These have to undergo phase I trials to prove safety and further trials to prove they are effective before they are allowed to be used. If proven to work, LBPs are certain to be classified as drugs, with specific health claims, indications, dosages, and side effects—just like any medication.

There are various LBPs already under development. One is a defined bacterial consortium of eight strains of commensal *C. difficile*, given orally at a daily dose of 8 billion CFU. The idea behind this novel formulation is that the benign forms of *C. diff* will specifically outcompete the pathogenic forms, allowing the rest of the bowel flora to return to normal without the use of either antibiotics or FMTs. Metagenomic analysis has demonstrated definite engraftment of these strains, and this was observed only in those who responded to treatment. The authors are pretty proud of their achievement, stating, "To our knowledge this is the first double blind placebo-controlled study to demonstrate efficacy with a defined bacterial consortium in any therapeutic indication." It's an exciting moment![45]

Another is a strain of the human vaginal bacilli *Lactobacillus crispatus*, specifically selected and shown to be effective for symptomatic bacterial vaginosis. Again, this is one of the very few practical applications of knowledge of the microbiome that is being translated into clinical practice and may well be coming soon to a practice near you.[46]

What Is the Supplement Paradox?

Fecal transplants, vaginal microbiome transplants, and certain novel probiotics really do appear to have proven effectiveness for specific conditions, in contrast to conventional probiotics, for which the evidence is very weak. At the end of the day, though, it almost doesn't matter. The supplement paradox informs us that no matter what the evidence says, people will continue to take them.

Decades of evidence shows that taking vitamins, minerals, and botanicals such as vitamin D, glucosamine, and echinacea makes no difference to people's health, or in some cases, actively causes harm. Of course, some vitamins and minerals really do help, but even these tend to be overused or used by healthy people. But all of this information makes no difference to the supplement market.

People are either unaware of these negative results, don't trust the scientific process, or perhaps simply find the results baffling. Supplements have entered the common consciousness as healthy, with over 50 percent of Americans having taken one supplement or another in the past month no matter what the evidence says.

In a similar way, as much as the evidence and the guidance point us away from probiotics as effective therapies, just as they do for supplements, probiotics continue to be extremely popular and are taken by many. The global probiotics market tells the same story. With a compound annual growth rate of over 9 percent, this market is set to be strong for the foreseeable future.

We could argue it almost doesn't matter; that probiotics mainly don't do any harm. We can almost admire the chutzpah of the probiotic advertising claims, promoting products using only "potentially misleading" health claims and somehow making us feel that we are doing ourselves good by buying their products. That is, until we hear of someone with a serious illness spending hundreds of dollars on a probiotic. They are hoping that the probiotic will save them. But we now know, that at worst, probiotics can kill and, at best, they have no effect.[47]

9

LOSS OF MICROBIOME DIVERSITY

What Do We Mean by Diversity?

The word "diversity" is a familiar word, known to us all. It implies variety; something composed of different elements or qualities; "a state of being diverse." But diversity does not just have its colloquial use. It also has a special scientific use too, relevant for analyzing the microbiome. Diversity is a key measure with respect to the microbiome, referring to the number or "richness" of microbial species in a sample. Because this concept is so important, analyzing it is not just left to chance or a few hyperbolic adjectives. It is measured as exactly as possible using statistical concepts, calculations, and formulae developed in the 1960s, and the terms "alpha diversity" and "beta diversity" are now used to express diversity in a specific way.[1]

In straightforward terms, alpha diversity refers to the number of species within one subunit—for example, the number of plant species within a swamp. For us, focusing specifically on microbiomes, this might be the number of different species of microbes found in one person's gut.

In contrast, beta diversity considers the species diversity in the whole landscape. It might compare the number of plant species next to a lake to the number of plant species next to a different lake a few miles away. For us, focusing on the microbiome, this measurement allows us to compare the variety of microbial species *between* people. A group of people living in a home together, say a family, would tend to have more similar sets of microbes in their intestines to each other than to those in the intestines of another family. We could then describe this as a lower beta diversity.

However, it has to be acknowledged that neither the colloquial meaning nor the scientific definition covers all the meanings of the word "diversity." Diversity, as we know, can refer to much more loaded political issues, a point squarely recognized by both American and English dictionary definitions, which start with the definition of diversity and then continue with "especially the practice or quality of including or involving people from a range of different social and ethnic backgrounds."

Involving people from a range of different backgrounds neatly sums up some of the preoccupations and direction of travel of microbiome research, which right from the start has been focused on contrasting microbiomes of people with differing diets, lifestyles, cultures, ethnicities, and nationalities to try and understand why we have the microbiomes that we have.

Is Research on the Microbiome Diverse Enough?

Metagenomic research on the microbiome started out with, as we know, the Human Microbiome Project, which centered on samples collected in large urban centers in America such as Houston, Texas, and St. Louis, Missouri. The key attribute of every one of those initial 242 subjects was that they had to be completely healthy. But apart from health, two other things were also specifically aimed for and achieved in initial subject choices: an equal sex ratio and "20% minority (racial and ethnic) participants." The initial analysis included subjects born all over the world, including Africa, Asia, Europe, the Middle East, and South America.[2]

Although the Human Microbiome Project started well, the ethnocultural diversity of microbiome research and whether it is diverse enough is a topic for debate, with some scientists arguing that we need "an improved understanding of the biological consequences of the construct of race and its function" and others saying that studies on race simply repeat outdated historical narratives.[3,4]

Others have complained that too much microbiome research has focused on Europe and America and not enough on the rest of the world, with only 3 percent focusing on subjects from Africa, for example.[5]

186 THE MICROBIOME

But metagenomic research is expensive, and each country has to consider this in their decisions about which health projects to fund and which scientific projects to engage with. As costs have reduced and technology improved, larger studies and in more populations have been undertaken, and there is now metagenomic research being undertaken in most countries of the world. Countries that can afford it have focused their projects on issues relevant to themselves, with researchers in Bangladesh and Cambodia, for example, focusing on issues such as severe malnutrition. Meanwhile, the National Institutes of Health, the Bill and Melinda Gates Foundation, and the European Union have rushed to fill the gap and help fund continuing research all around the world.

Studies from around the world are important and lend credence to certain findings; when we find the same vaginal microbiome in Japan as we do in Sweden or the same neonatal bifidobacteria in Gambia as in Brazil, it adds weight to the importance of that microbe, to the evidence for coevolution, and the importance of vertical transmission.

Right from the start, it has been obvious that there is a real variety in stool microbiomes between different populations, between developed and developing countries, and between urban and rural areas. Microbiome researchers have been keen to compare samples from different populations in different countries of the world and not just focus on Western countries. Some of the most interesting samples have been obtained from people living rather unique lifestyles, such as hunter-gatherers.

Because of the power differentials between scientific researchers and these communities, there has been a certain amount of tension associated with these data-gathering exercises.[6] Some researchers have famously crossed scientific boundaries in their interactions with certain communities, with one researcher, Jeff D. Leach, infamously using a turkey baster to give himself a fecal transplant from a member of a hunter-gatherer community, and anthropologist Kenneth Good actually marrying a young girl from the isolated Yanomami tribe that he was studying and having three children. Amazingly, his son David Good, brought up in the Western world, eventually returned to the Amazon as a microbiome researcher himself and was able to make contact with his mother and extended family.[7]

How Is the Microbiome Different between People in Urban Areas Compared to Rural?

It has become clear that overall, people who live in urban areas have many fewer microbial species in their gut microbiomes (a markedly reduced alpha diversity) than people who live in traditional rural areas, such as subsistence farmers. Although the dominant gut bacteria in both populations are typically non-sporing anaerobes (*Bacteroides* and *Bifidobacteria*), urban specimens often contain up to thirty times more *Bacteroides* (bacteria known for digesting protein and fats). In contrast, people who live in traditional rural communities tend to have a more diverse set of microbes, typically containing more *Prevotella* (bacteria known for digesting plant carbohydrates) as well as a higher alpha diversity. This is nicely demonstrated in an early exploratory study that compared the fecal microbiomes of children living in Florence, Italy, to children from the Mossi ethnic group living in Boulpon, a small village in Burkina Faso, Western Africa.

Being brought up in Florence in 2010 couldn't have been more different than being brought up in Boulpon. As well as having many remarkable monuments and art galleries, Florence is a place of apartments, tarmac, and Vespa mopeds zipping around. In contrast, Boulpon is quiet, small, and surrounded by fields with traditional termite mud huts and unpaved paths.

The children from Burkina Faso were eating millet grain ground by their mothers on a traditional grinding stone, as well as sorghum, black-eyed peas, and vegetables, but hardly any meat—usually chicken or, if it was the rainy season, termites. This compared to the children in Florence, who had a typical Western diet, high in animal protein, sugar, starch, and fat. The calorie intake was also strikingly different: 996 kilocalories per day for the Burkina Faso children and 1,512 kilocalories per day for the Italian children. Typical fiber intake was 14.2 grams per day in Burkina Faso compared to 5.6 grams per day in an EU diet.

As we would expect, microbiome analyses of these children's stools show a lot more *Bacteroides* in the Italian children and, in comparison, a lot more *Prevotella* and overall higher species richness in the Burkina

188 THE MICROBIOME

Faso children. The Burkina Faso children also had a corkscrew or spiral-shaped spirochaetes microbe detectable in their samples, a microbe called *Treponema succinifaciens*, completely absent in the Italian children.

The lives of these two groups of children—their environment, their food, ethnicity, sanitation, access to medicines, geography, and climate—are all so different that it is hard to know which factor has caused these differences in their gut microbes or if, in fact, it is a combination of several. This was an early study on the subject, an exploratory study, and the researchers suggested the main causal difference was diet. However, they go further, suggesting that the people living in this village "live in an environment that still resembles that of Neolithic subsistence farmers," and that the diversity of their microbiomes represents "a goldmine," both for further research and the potential development of novel probiotics.[8]

The authors, as we have seen, don't make assumptions about the lifestyle of the Boulpon villagers and carefully describe their living conditions and diet in detail. But whether this resembles the lifestyle of Neolithic farmers is difficult to know. If it did, then these samples could represent a sort of time travel into the past, an almost historical investigation: an idea that has really captured the imagination of some microbiome researchers. And if a rural African village could inform us on Neolithic microbiomes 10,000 years ago, then could samples from hunter-gatherers inform us of a time even earlier, a time before farming and static living, stretching to when modern humans were first recognized over 100,000 years ago?

Do Hunter-Gatherers Have a Distinctive Microbiome?

Although it is hard not to get carried away, it is important not to romanticize people living a traditional subsistence rural or hunter-gatherer lifestyle or assume they are living just like Neolithic farmers or hunter-gatherers did thousands of years ago. These are modern people living in modern times just as we all are, not throwbacks to early humans. Nor is there a standard rural or hunter-gatherer diet; each group has a different diet according to where they live in the world. Many live a transitional lifestyle that includes Western foods, modern medicines, and factory-made clothes being used daily, weekly, less frequently, or never, depending on the choices or habits of that specific group or individual.[9]

However, in spite of these cautionary approaches, interest in the stool and skin microbiomes of hunter-gatherers remains high. It is palpably obvious how different their lifestyles are from most of the rest of the world; they are in constant contact with the natural environment, they often live in temporary self-built shelters using natural materials, and their diets are varied with a minimal amount of processed foods or farmed grains. There are more hunter-gatherer groups in the world than perhaps we might have expected or ever heard of. Groups studied with respect to the microbiome include the Hadza people in Tanzania, the Yanomami in Brazil, the BaAka rainforest hunter-gatherers from Central Africa, the Agta in the Philippines, and the Chepang in the Himalayas, but there are many others. One of the first studies to draw everyone's attention to the marked microbiome differences found between these populations was one that compared urban families in the cities of St. Louis and Philadelphia in America to a rural community in Malawi, Southeast Africa, and a group of Ghahibo Amerindians in the Amazonas State of Venezuela—three places and lifestyles that couldn't be more in contrast. A reduced species richness was immediately apparent both from rural to urban, as we have already seen, but also from hunter-gatherer to rural: 1,600 OTUs (operational taxonomic units; approximately equivalent to the number of microbial species per person) in hunter-gatherer samples, 1,400 in rural samples, and 1,200 in the urban samples.[10]

One group of hunter-gatherers that has been particularly studied is the Hadza hunter-gatherer population, and some species found in the Hadza are simply not found in urban samples, ever. They have appeared to have simply vanished or perhaps even become extinct. This lost group of microbes is designated by the authors as "VANISH" taxa (Volatile and/or Associated Negatively with Industrialised Societies of Humans taxa) and includes microbes from the *Prevoltellaceae*, *Succinovibrionaceae*, *Paraprevotellaceae*, and *Spirochaetaceae* families. They are found in high levels in hunter-gatherer populations right across the world but rarely or never in urban populations. They too include *Treponema succinifaciens*, the spiral-shaped bacterium that we have already come across in the Burkina Faso children although the significance of this organism is unknown.[11,12]

The one set of hunter-gatherer groups that bucks this trend is the Canadian Arctic people, who, with a non-tropical lifestyle and a high-meat and low-fiber diet, have a similar microbiome profile and diversity to people living in the urban center of Montreal, Canada. They show the typical high *Bacteroides* and low *Prevotella* profile of an urban or Westernized population. Like the Yanomami, the Hadza, and all the other groups, the transitional nature and progressive Westernization of this group means, however, that all of their diets are changing rapidly or indeed have already changed.[13]

What Is the Cause of These Differences in Microbiome Diversity?

The people involved in these early studies have such contrasting lifestyles that it's hard to work out what is causing their marked differences and steep decrease in diversity: the diet, the latitude, the environment, the housing, or a whole host of other possibilities. But by contrasting groups of people with the same ethnic background, living in the same latitude, the same geographical location, and even consuming essentially the same diet but with just one or two carefully delineated differences in lifestyles, it is possible to iron out some possibilities and work out in more detail what exactly could be causing these differences.

Irish travelers represent 1 percent of the population of Ireland and were granted separate ethnic status in 2017 in recognition of their distinct culture and history, but genetically they are very similar to the settled Irish population. They have a similar diet to the rest of the population and obviously live in the same country with the same natural environment and the same weather. But from a lifestyle point of view, they are very different. They have very large families (mean sibling count 9.8 compared to 1.38 for the general population), a high animal ownership (mean 68.6 percent compared to 42 percent estimated for the general population), and often live in close confinement in mobile or trailer homes, although changes in law in the last twenty years have meant that most travelers now live on static sites.

When stool samples are compared between Irish travelers and the settled population, their gut diversity reveals a very distinct separation, midway between hunter-gatherers and industrialized populations. This is not because of their nomadic lifestyle, which is mainly not nomadic anymore, but perhaps is because of the domestic conditions associated with nomadism: being outside more and the "particularly close living quarters that favour horizontal microbial dispersal . . . accentuated by large family sizes." Animal ownership must also play its part.[14]

Another attempt to delineate key causes of altered diversity focuses on three groups living in the Himalayas: one with a hunter-gatherer lifestyle, one that has recently transitioned to farming, and one that has been farming for over 200 years. Again, this eliminates factors related to ethnicity, latitude, the environment, diet, sanitation, and access to medical care, as well as giving us a sense of the time course. These changes in lifestyle have also led to decreased diversity, the microbes altering from a typical hunter-gatherer set including *Treponema* and *Ruminobacter* to a typical rural farming type set, indicating rapid change within a generation. In addition, the water source and use of solid cooking fuel used by each group made a significant difference.[15]

But change can be quicker even than a generation. Stools from new US immigrants originally from Thailand and now living in Minnesota demonstrate a rapid loss of diversity within months, including loss of native strains, loss of *Prevotella*, and emerging dominance of *Bacteroides*, even when diets remained distinct from the rest of the population.[16]

It appears that the cause of reduced alpha diversity in modern urban populations is probably multifactorial and not just diet-related. Ethnicity is probably not a key factor, but diet and fiber intake, the water source, built living quarters, reduced contact with the natural environment, and reduced contact with animals must all play their part. In the close-set, highly populated urban conurbations of modern life, we have learned by bitter experience to adhere strongly to the principles of cleanliness, hygiene, sewage engineering, and waste disposal in order to avoid the high mortality from infectious disease that we saw in the cities of the 19th and 20th centuries, and this has necessarily had an impact on our microbiomes.

192 THE MICROBIOME

Can Archaeological Samples Tell Us about Microbiome Diversity in the Past?

So far, we have tried to use rural and hunter-gatherer populations as a window into the past to try to visualize how microbial diversity has changed over time and work out what factors may have caused that change. However, a better way of tracking microbial changes in the human gut through history may be to look at *actual* samples from the past, from mummified bodies, ancient archaeological sites, or even from fossils.

Well-desiccated 1,000-year-old DNA tends to fragment somewhat; but even so, certain familiar bacteria can be identified. Samples taken from the colon of a natural mummy found in the Colombian Andes and dated to 1100 AD show various microbes, including our old favorite, *Bacteroidetes*. Unfortunately, the predominance of *Clostridium* also picked up probably just reflects that bacteria's temporary overgrowth after death and suggests that the consortium of bacteria found in this mummy is unlikely to represent a typical microbiome of the time.[17]

Attempts have been made to analyze archaeological samples, and it has been found possible to extract DNA from coprolites (fossilized stool) thought to be up to 2,000 years old. Like the Colombian mummy, the DNA is very fragmented and suffers from risks of contamination by modern microbes. *Callidusccus callidus* and *Treponema succinifaciens* were identified, along with several other microbes, but not enough for a full description of an ancient stool microbiome and certainly not enough to tell us about any change in diversity.[18]

Crossing species and stretching back 50,000 years are stool samples from Neanderthal sites: tiny phosphatic coprolites, just millimeters across, representing the oldest known positive identification of human fecal matter. Amazingly, these too reveal a few bacteria, including well-known gut commensals such as *Bifidobacterium* and *Faecalibacterium*, bacterial lineages probably shared between us and Neanderthals.[19]

Fascinating as these studies are, they have only really confirmed the existence of ancient microbiota, not cast a light on the diversity of the prehistoric human microbiome.

Can Samples from Other Mammals Show How Our Microbiome Evolved?

Comparing ourselves to our nearest living hominid relatives and other mammals can give us a much more complete window on the past and how our microbes evolved with us, meaning we don't need to work so hard with these fragmented or possibly contaminated microbial DNA samples to study changes in diversity or the evolutionary origins of our microbiome.

Samples from great apes such as gorillas, chimpanzees, and bonobos reveal a shared gut microbial heritage—a family tree of microbes whose divergence from each other and from us exactly matches known genetic divergence times, with a last common ancestor approximately 6 million years ago. Familiar bacteria are present but in different proportions. *Bacteroides* species are five times more common in humans than in apes, whereas the archaeon *Methanobrevibacter*, which is good at digesting really tough plant fiber, has undergone a fivefold reduction.

As well as an overall loss of whole bacterial families in humans compared to great apes, there is also an overall loss of diversity, with fewer species found in humans than in great apes, even in humans living a hunter-gatherer lifestyle. Where the average number of bacterial genera per individual is about eighty-five in wild apes, there are only about seventy per individual in hunter-gatherers, compared to sixty in rural Malawi and fifty-five in the urban United States. This steady drop could imply that lower bacterial diversity is normal for humans. "Consistent with the known dietary shifts that occurred during human evolution, taxa that have been associated with the digestion of animal food stuffs have risen in relative abundance in the human gut microbiome, whereas taxa that have been associated with the digestion of plant-based diets have become less prominent."[20]

If we then look at other non-human primates, including purely leaf-eating or florivorous species, and indeed other animals such as meat eaters, omnivores, and herbivores, we can infer past evolutionary processes that reach right back to the dawn of mammals, 66 million years ago. Although the evolutionary history of microbes is a large and fascinating topic and can be taken back much further than this, this is the furthest date back in time we will dare to consider here.[21]

194 THE MICROBIOME

The gut microbiomes of each mammalian species can be readily distinguished from each other based on their microbial compositions alone. Some scientists claim that they can describe a "core mammalian microbiome" with more closely related species demonstrating more similar communities of microbes.[22]

It is immediately obvious from these comparisons that herbivores routinely have a higher microbial diversity than omnivores and carnivores; herbivores are dependent on microbes to ferment the cellulose and resistant starches of the tough grasses and leaves that they eat in a way that omnivores and carnivores are not. To enable this fermentation, herbivores have evolved a much more complex and enlarged gut than other animals and developed a much slower transit time. In contrast, carnivores have a relatively simple gut, a fast transit time, and a much-reduced bacterial diversity. Omnivores, of which we as humans are one, come somewhere in the middle, depending on how much protein is contained in our diets.

But microbial diversity is not just a factor of diet. Where animals have evolved from carnivores but adapted to a leaf-eating diet, they retain the simpler gut and reduced microbial diversity consistent with their heritage. Red pandas and giant pandas are fascinating examples of this, as are the foliage-eating primates such as Colobus and Langur monkeys. Conversely, where omnivores have evolved into meat-eaters only, like whales and dolphins, they too demonstrate a loss of bacteria taxa but also an increased divergence rate.

The gut environment, as we discussed in the gut chapter, can be thought of as an open ecosystem and is subject to a constant influx of microbial colonizers. But it is also a curated environment, and only certain taxa can survive the temperatures, fluids, acids, and so on. Many species of animal, particularly herbivores, obtain their microbes from their environment and then curate the microbial species depending on their internal anatomical architecture. But the distinct microbiomes that some mammals display also imply widespread horizontal transmission within family and social groups, and perhaps also sometimes some vertical transmission from mother to baby.

Do the Changes in Our Microbiome Diversity Impact Our Health?

It is not yet clear whether decreased microbiome diversity is normal for humans or might be having an effect on our health. But it has been observed that a certain class of disease has been rising in some populations as standards of living, such as access to clean water, food security, and reduced overcrowding, have improved. Sometimes described as "diseases of the affluent," these include a wide variety: vascular diseases such as heart disease, type 2 diabetes, and hypertension; atopic diseases such as eczema, asthma, hay fever, and allergy; and a smorgasbord of others, including appendicitis, inflammatory bowel disease, and multiple sclerosis. These have been seen rising first in developed countries as standards of living have improved over time and then in developing countries as standards of living improve there. They are also often seen rising in groups of immigrants that have come from developing countries to developed countries.

The increase of heart disease, type 2 diabetes, and hypertension is well known in immigrants and is reasonably attributed to reduced activity and eating too much food. But the increasing incidence of other diseases of affluence is less easily explained. Why should the incidence of asthma or appendicitis increase? Could these increases be attributed to the rapid recent changes to our microbiomes, particularly the decrease in diversity?

In some ways, reassuringly, humans appear to fit in with the evolutionary history of gut microbiomes in mammals. We have a gut microbe diversity typical for an omnivore. We display a simplified gut and a reduction of plant-digesting species and loss of taxa as we trend more and more towards eating energy-dense foods such as animal protein and fat. Even the recent speeding up of microbe divergence is consistent with other mammals who have followed the same diet trajectory. Those of us with the most microbial species in our guts (hunter-gatherers) still demonstrate a marked drop in diversity compared to other primates, implying that our loss of diversity is normal for humans.

However, with urbanization going hand-in-hand with sanitation just in the last 200 years, and the advent of modern medicine and highly processed foods in the last 100, there has been a demonstrable sea change in

196   THE MICROBIOME

our environments. Multiple factors in modern daily life have significantly reduced our exposure to different microbes, and as we have seen, study after study highlights the marked reduction in microbial diversity of people living in cities. Important public health measures have been introduced deliberately in the dense urban conurbations of cities to reduce our exposure to microbes, aimed at reducing our exposure to pathogens, and they have worked. Our life expectancy has been rising all this time as deaths from infectious disease have fallen. But has this reduced exposure to microbes led to an increase in other diseases?

Although not so well known today, appendicitis was for a long time regarded as a disease of the affluent. It was apparently so rare in developing countries that in East Africa in the 1920s it was said that only those who spoke English developed it. India was another country where it was regarded as unusual. "Hallilay (1924) cited many examples of the rare incidence of appendicitis in Indians, with the exception of members of the upper classes who had adopted many Western customs."[23] Although it is difficult to accurately measure the rise in appendicitis as access to surgery and diagnostic criteria have changed, it is clear that the incidence of appendicitis in Western countries increased through the first part of the 20th century, peaking in the 1950s before declining.

The incidence of allergies, hay fever, eczema, and asthma has also increased, particularly hay fever, which we will focus on for a moment. This increase in hay fever was first observed and commented on as early as 1873. Charles Harrison Blackley (1820–1900), an English doctor who himself suffered from hay fever, tracked the number of publications on the subject, using this as a surrogate for its incidence. In his book *Experimental Researches on the Causes and Nature of Catarrhus Aestivus*, he describes how, after the condition was first described in 1819, nothing was published for ten years. Then eighteen cases were described, and after that, there was another ten-year hiatus before publications and case studies gradually became more common, concluding, "It would seem that there are now a greater number of cases to be met with than there were formerly."

With great humility, Blackley points out that in hay fever "the non-occurrence of sequelae of a serious character, seem to offer opportunities for safe experimentation such as are rarely found in any other complaint." This aspect of hay fever encouraged him to experiment on himself. For over a decade, he exposed himself to heat, dust, hayfields, changes of weather, strong perfumes, and over 160 different types of plant pollen, finally concluding that hay fever resulted from a combination of factors: both from "some peculiarity of the constitution" plus contact with pollen. He attributes the rising incidence of hay fever that he observed to several factors: the increase in hay farming, the marked increase in population evident at the time, and the increased proportion of those living in cities.[24]

"Hay fever is said to be an aristocratic disease" he says, "a disorder almost wholly confined to the educated classes." He concludes, "There can be no doubt that that condition of the nervous system which mental training generates is one which is especially favourable to the development of [hay fever]." Of course, his conclusion that hay fever is caused by being educated seems laughable to us today, but it is a salutary lesson for us measuring various weak associations between gut microbiomes and different diseases about how wrong we can be. The one thing he and all of the other writers on hay fever agreed on was that farmers never got it. Nobody knew why this was. Some said it was because of their strong constitutions, others their constant exposure to pollens, and still others that it was something inherent in their healthy outdoor lifestyle. However, the idea that people brought up on farms are in some way protected from allergies and atopy is an idea that scientists have returned to many times since Blackley's book was published, and to which we will come back later in the chapter.

Asthma is another atopic disease that has been increasing in incidence in the last century. Unlike hay fever, asthma has had a longer history. As a word, it was used by the ancient Greeks apparently to describe a sort of shortness of breath; someone could have "asthma" just before an important battle, perhaps depicting the kind of breathlessness more related to getting hyped up or angry rather than referring to a specific illness or what we would call asthma today. Although there appear to be possible attempts to describe asthma in the Middle Ages, it is a book called *A Treatise of the Asthma* by John Floyer, published in 1698, that contains one of the earliest descriptions of asthma as we would recognize it today. Floyer is another physician who suffered from the condition that he wrote about: "I have fuffered under the Tyranny of the Afthma, at leaft, Thirty years; and therefore think my felf to be fully informed in the Hiftory of that Difeafe."

He specifically focuses on "periodic asthma" and correctly describes this as constriction of the bronchia, wheezing, and difficulty breathing. "If this difficulty [of breath] be by the constriction of the bronchia 'tis properly the periodic asthma: and if the constriction be great, it is with wheezing; but if less the wheezing is not so evident." He also describes the diurnal nature of the condition (worse in the early hours of the morning or at night and better during the day) in what feels like a firsthand account: "At first waking about one or two of the clock in the night, the fit of asthma more evidently begins, the asthmatic is immediately necessitated to rise out of his bed."

He says, "I cannot remember the first occasion of my asthma but have been told that it was a cold when I first went to school." He concludes, "As my asthma is not hereditary from my ancestors, I thank God, neither of my two sons are inclined to it, who are now past the age in which it seized me."[25]

Since Floyer first clearly described the nature of asthma, just like hay fever and appendicitis, it too has become more prevalent in the Western world. Again, changes in diagnostic indicators make it hard to compare figures, but since the 1950s, the incidence of asthma in the United Kingdom has risen from 1.4 percent to 2.3 percent in the 1960s and 9.3 percent in the 1980s before finally leveling off at 11.6 percent of six-year-olds today, a change mirrored across the world. In fact, there has been a documented increase in the incidence of all atopic diseases across the world; the incidence of hay fever, asthma, eczema, and allergies have all increased and then leveled off. The question is, why?[26]

What Is the Hygiene Hypothesis?

The hygiene hypothesis is the idea that as our living conditions have improved, with access to toilets, clean water, and kitchen hygiene, we are missing out on contact with ordinary microbes. This means that our immune systems are not being "trained" properly, and they then overreact or react to our own bodies, leading to the increase in the rate of allergic diseases. This broad failure of immunoregulation is also thought to be the cause of the increase in conditions such as Crohn's disease and multiple sclerosis. Many scientists attribute the increase in atopy and other diseases of affluence to the "hygiene hypothesis."

The earliest mention of the hygiene hypothesis was in a paper that linked rates of appendicitis to access to a bathroom. This was a large and powerful study based on 5,362 British children assessed in 1946, which found that a household without a bathroom was associated with a reduced relative risk of appendicitis (0.7). Lack of a hot water system and shared use of a kitchen were also associated with a reduced risk (0.9). Barker notes that his "findings support the hygiene hypothesis. This suggests that as hygiene improved young children began to escape infection and thereby became more vulnerable to appendicitis when exposed to infections in later childhood and early adult life."[27]

However, it was David P. Strachan, lecturer in epidemiology at the London School of Hygiene and Tropical Medicine (and with a self-avowed love of alliteration), who popularized the term. His paper "Hay Fever, Hygiene, and Household Size" was another powerful study based on large numbers of British patients, and his results added weight to Barker's theory. Strachan looked at the incidence of asthma in over 17,000 children and showed that there was a clear and indisputable link with family size. Those with four or more older siblings had an incidence of asthma of 2.6 percent, only a quarter of the rate of those without older siblings (10 percent). The number of younger siblings made no difference. Data on eczema told the same story: less than half the rate in a child with four older siblings (2.8 percent) than with none (6.1 percent).[28]

These findings, that older siblings were protective for atopy, were found again and again in repeated studies, but were difficult to explain. Initially, it was thought that a decreased rate of childhood respiratory infections such as coughs and colds was the problem, but further research did not support this conclusion.

Allergic diseases appeared to be prevented not by high levels of respiratory infections in childhood but by "unhygienic contact with older siblings," as Strachan puts it, linking with Barker's evidence that reduced access to hygiene protected children from appendicitis. "Over the past century declining family size, improvements in household amenities and higher standards of personal cleanliness have reduced the opportunity for cross infection in young families. This may have resulted in more widespread clinical expression of atopic disease, emerging earlier in wealthier people, as seems to have occurred for hay fever" (see note 28).

Building on this research in the 1990s, large studies across Europe looked at the incidence of allergic disease in children brought up on farms. The PASTURE group (Protection Against Allergy—Study in Rural Environments) was based on 1,000 children recruited in Germany, Austria, Switzerland, and Finland. There was also the ALEX group (the Allergy and Endotoxin study), the PARSIFAL study (Prevention of Allergy—Risk Factors for Sensitization Related to Farming and Anthroposophic Lifestyle), and many others returning to Blackley's original idea that farmers don't get atopy.

As well as children with older siblings being protected, these studies showed that children who live on farms are also protected. However, if a child then moves to the city, especially if they are below a certain age (five years for asthma, older for other illnesses), the protection is lost. The farm effect is independent of the sibling effect and is remarkably reproducible across populations and continents. The effects are strong, with children on farms having about half the risk of developing hay fever compared to a city child.[29]

The microbes these children are exposed to—on the farm, in the cowsheds, and in other animal sheds—are found in their nasal passages, on their skin, in the dust in their rooms, and even on their beds. "Children also bring their microbial exposures into the indoor environment, where microorganisms and their compounds settle in floor and mattress dust. Thus, mattress dust can be regarded as a reservoir that reflects an individual's long-term microbial exposure in indoor and outdoor environments." As well as being protected by growing up on a farm or by having older siblings, children who have pets are also protected, as are those who drink unpasteurized milk, those who are weaned earlier, and those attending daycare.[30]

Although drinking unpasteurized cow's milk is definitely not routinely recommended due to the risks of food-based infection, the idea that constant exposure to multiple microbes is protective against atopic disease fits with all of the evidence. That multiple factors all appear to be protective indicates that there must be some interplay between these protective elements, which probably involve both the airway, the nose, and the gut. It appears the more microbes we are exposed to, the better, and many papers conclude that we need microbes to "train" our immune system.

Immunology is a large and important discipline that we cannot do more than touch on here, but of course, we know that the immune system is not "trained" in the way we like to train our staff or our army personnel. We know that the cells in the innate immune system are born automatically able to recognize the foreign-looking material of bacterial cell walls and need no "training" to be able to identify or attack them. Meanwhile, the cells of the adaptive immune system are being made in their millions throughout our lives, each one unique and each one able to attack a different antigen, even antigens that do not exist as yet. But before any adaptive immune cell is released into the body to get to work and defend us, it is checked, and any cell that is found to react to "self" (and this includes over 99 percent of them) is eliminated, killed by murderous guard cells specifically detailed for the job: as we said, not "training" in the way we like to see in our national institutions, but certainly an effective system. Somehow, constant low-level exposure to varied microbes must be helping this process to work properly. Many detailed immunological mechanisms have been suggested for this protective effect, but the exact mechanism has so far not been agreed upon.

The loss of exposure to ordinary microbes that we have experienced through the different factors that we have discussed—smaller families, reduced overcrowding, sanitation, reduced contact with animals, reduced contact with the natural world, food processing, clean water, sewage engineering, modern medical care, access to cesareans, and in particular, the use of antibiotics—has clearly had a recent and real impact on the number of species of microbes found in the typical human. This reduction is arguably over and above the natural tendency of reduced diversity seen in omnivores approaching a more meat-led diet. This delineation of a recent and sudden reduction in microbial diversity has led to urgent and panicked conclusions by some scientists: that we are losing our microbes, that we have had irreversible microbial extinctions, and that this will lead to an epidemic of allergy and other immune-based diseases. Described as an "ominous trend," some say that our microbial communities may no longer be compatible with our human biology. "It is our opinion that aspects of our microbial identity have gone extinct and that this extinction results in a mismatch between our recently adapted microbiota and our more slowly adapting human genome."[31]

It is clear that there really has been a decrease in human gut microbial diversity and that there really has been a real increase in some diseases of affluence, and this may be explained by the hygiene hypothesis (although it doesn't quite explain the plateauing or even decrease that we have seen in some diseases of affluence). Whether or not the decreases in our gut microbial diversity are in any way causal is unclear. It may just serve as a proxy for measuring the microbial diversity in the environment around us.

But even if a decrease in human microbiome diversity is responsible for an increase in atopy, it would still be very important not to lose a sense of perspective. If the goal is to increase human life expectancy (and at the rate we are overrunning the planet, this might not always be our goal), but if it is, then all of the above measures, but especially sanitation and food and water hygiene, have significantly reduced our mortality and morbidity from infectious diseases. Think of all of those children who had to suffer and die from tuberculosis of the gastrointestinal tract before the advent of bacteriology and public health eliminated the carriage of tuberculosis from our cattle and their milk. Measures such as having an emergency cesarean birth, although undoubtedly having an impact (hopefully temporary) on the newborn baby's exposure to microbes, will have certainly reduced the chance of their mother dying, for example, from obstructed labor. Most children born by cesarean are okay; it is true that on average they have slightly more asthma than those born vaginally.

Those of us living with the least amount of interference from public health measures and all the other aspects of a Western lifestyle—today's hunter-gatherers—have a life expectancy at birth of twenty-one to thirty-seven years, reflecting their very high rate of infant and childhood mortality from infectious disease. We can compare this to life expectancy at birth in Europe, on average eighty years, which has gone up even in our lifetime. Should a hunter-gatherer finally reach adulthood, he or she can expect to live until seventy-six but will still tend to die of infectious illnesses (55 percent) and violence (17 percent), although admittedly heart attacks and strokes are rare. In the United States, in contrast, about 3 percent of deaths are caused by infectious disease, usually influenza, pneumonia, or sepsis.

Can We Rewild Our Microbiomes?

Although public health measures have overall improved our life expectancy and reduced our exposure to pathogens, they have also reduced our exposure to many benign microbes that we may, in fact, benefit from. As Blaser says, "the remarkable aspect of vertebrate life is not that we respond to pathogens, but that we so easily tolerate the overwhelming numbers of commensal microorganisms that we host." But it's not just that we tolerate them; it appears that to avoid atopic disease, we need them—small continual doses of them. Both to be in contact with them with our hands and skin, on our food and water to make contact with our gut, and through our nasal passages and lungs by breathing them in (see note 31).[32]

On the other hand, can't we have both? Can't we both avoid infectious diseases through modern public health measures and get plenty of contact with the natural world? This would enable us to both avoid infectious diseases and at the same time avoid asthma and other atopic diseases. The children being brought up on farms, in large families, with animals, or in contact with nature suggest that we can. They have both avoided infectious disease and have a lower chance of developing atopic disease.

What is obvious is that both pathogens and ordinary microbes are spread in the same way—through close contact, overcrowding, large families, reduced access to hygiene, sewage, dirty water, and so on. No one wants to go back to the epidemics of typhoid, scarlet fever, and cholera that we suffered in the 19th and 20th centuries, nor do we want to encounter sick

204 THE MICROBIOME

bugs if we can avoid them, or food poisoning if we don't handle raw meat correctly.

However, if we can avoid allergic diseases with straightforward and safe measures, then perhaps we can both have our cake and eat it too. We want to tread a delicate line: on the one hand, avoiding serious infections and, on the other hand, reducing the chance of atopic diseases and other diseases related to an imbalance of the immune system.

Many of us already achieve this balance, this best of two worlds. Many people are generally healthy; neither at risk from most epidemic infections because of strong public health measures, and lucky enough to have avoided asthma, eczema, hay fever, appendicitis, inflammatory bowel disease, and multiple sclerosis. Others may have a family history of atopy but are inadvertently following lifestyle measures that allow them to be in contact with a variety of microbes; maybe they are the youngest in the family, or happen to live on a farm, or own pets, and so have personally avoided developing eczema or asthma.

Some things are hard to change. Where we may have been born by cesarean, bottle-fed, or had multiple courses of antibiotics as a child (perhaps for life-threatening infections), is too late to alter now. But nor should we unduly worry about these things, as we always have plenty of other chances to come into contact with microbes and top up our microbiomes.

To consciously increase our daily contact with microbes, contact with the natural environment would seem to be a good place to start. Gardening, sitting on grass, handling wood, and touching trees in the forest; all of these activities are pleasant and healthy for other reasons. Exercise and green spaces are good for our overall fitness levels and keep us in good spirits, as well as having the benefit of keeping us in daily contact with normal microbes. Pet ownership or contact with animals is nice but doesn't suit everyone. However, where people have pets or own animals, they can be confident that that daily contact is another nice way to increase their microbial contacts and microbiome variety.

Dietary measures, however, are within everyone's reach, and a lot has been talked about diets that are good for our "friendly bacteria," in particular by eating a variety of foods. Some sources suggest aiming for a certain number of different plant-based foods each week to both increase the number of different sorts of microbes that we consume on the surface of each food type, but also to nurture a larger variety of microbes inside our gut. A varied diet is important for many reasons: to obtain dietary nutrients, for enjoyment, and for company. Perhaps we can now add that it may contribute to improving our daily exposure to the wide variety of microbes we appear to benefit from.[33]

We have already discussed the importance of fiber in our diet and the microbes that start to digest our gut mucus if they don't have enough fiber. That advice still holds, and a good fiber intake would also be achieved by eating a wide variety of plants, hitting two birds with one stone (not literally). Of course, there is plenty of other excellent advice about food to consider, not necessarily related to the gut microbiome, such as taking time to eat and focusing on the food, both to enjoy it fully and to notice straight away when we are 80% satisfied so that we can stop eating. Most of all, trying and trying every day not to eat too much, which in our world of excess and delicious food is always a difficult thing. Even the Hadza hunter-gatherers, although they eat plenty of fiber and a variety of foods, if given the choice, would only eat meat and honey.

So-called Paleolithic diets involve eating vegetables, fruits, nuts, seeds, eggs, fish, and lean meat while excluding grains, dairy products, and sugar (all foods we have developed through farming) and appear, at first glance, to be the perfect healthy diet, offering both variety, plenty of vegetables, high fiber, and avoiding sugar and carbohydrates. Samples taken from people who have switched to a Paleolithic diet indeed show a marked increase in bowel microbiome diversity, almost matching the gut microbes of hunter-gatherers.[34]

But although the gut microbiome can be quickly transformed within months or even days of a change in diet or a trip to a wild holiday destination, it's important to point out that gut microbial diversity is only a surrogate for health. Long-term trials would have to be performed to see whether a measure like this made any difference to, for example, longevity, or rates of asthma, or incidence of inflammatory bowel disease, or any other meaningful measure of health. Measuring gut diversity is simple, but it is

206 THE MICROBIOME

only one measurement of the microbiome, and an increase in gut diversity does not mean that someone is suddenly healthy.[35]

What Will Future Human Microbiomes Look Like?

It is to be hoped that, armed with this evolving information, our microbiomes will once again improve in diversity as we improve the variety of foods we eat and try to make contact with nature, earth, plants, and animals a part of our daily routine, to tread that delicate balance between keeping our microbiomes in perfect working order while avoiding pathogens and disease.

But what if the opposite happened, and a dystopian future saw us confined to our homes in small groups for weeks on end with only processed foods available? Amazingly, this sort of life has already been modeled. The NASA space program back in 2010 recognized that the crew of any long-term space mission would carry their microbiome with them and be isolated for many days. Any perturbations of their gut microbiomes would be difficult to fix and have unknown health implications. It is remarkable that, as well as considering every other measurable parameter of a long-term space mission—such as mental health, activity levels, and nutritional intake—the NASA scientists should take the time to consider the astronauts' gut microbiomes. However, they did. They undertook to study them, to take regular samples before, during, and after missions, and to make recommendations for future space projects.

To practice for the two-year journey to Mars, NASA conceived the Mars500 project. In this exercise, they confined six astronauts for 520 days in a mock spacecraft. Just like on a real mission, their only foods were in dehydrated packets and fully processed, their drinking water constantly recycled, they had limited hygiene regimes, and their only contact was with each other.

This experiment was repeated with the Hawaii Space Exploration Analog and Simulation IV in 2015, when six crew members lived for 365 days in a Martian outpost mock-up habitat; a spherical-shaped dome, 36 feet (11 meters) in diameter, located on the barren slopes of a volcano.[36]

Samples of stool, skin, and environmental samples from these closed biodomes showed that each crew member's microbial diversity continued to be as high as when they started, with microbiomes becoming slightly more similar between crew members over time. The majority returned to their usual pattern within six months of the mission ending; healthy.

So we end our journey where we started it—with a vision of those large transparent biodomes that perhaps may one day be used on a Mars mission and the tiny microbiomes within the humans inside them.

CONCLUSION

We have come on a challenging journey through this book, visualizing the complexity of the microbiome, traveling through different microbiomes of the body—including the gut, the skin, and the brain—and understanding the techniques that allow us to see into the microbial world. But there are topics we have not focused on: the mouth, the nose, internal organs such as the liver, and, in particular, the eye and the lung. A more detailed chapter on the eye or the lung would be fascinating to delve into, but these are hot topics in a fast-developing area, and there is no consensus here as yet with regard to microbiomes. Some scientists believe that these areas harbor microbiomes too, albeit at low levels, but the consensus is growing that, in fact, in these instances the microbiome is "dynamic," here one moment and not the next, being constantly dealt with by our immune systems.[1]

Even the definition of the word "microbiome" has been a contentious and evolving issue, as we have seen, and ideas about "dynamic" microbiomes in the lung perhaps tell us that the definition may still evolve further.[2] As well as considering both the microbes and the biome, perhaps the definition should also mention that a true microbiome cannot be just a chance smattering of microbes found in a discrete anatomical area but implies that microbes are living there in significant numbers and replicating at a rate exceeding loss due to death or excretion: a stable association, not just an extermination.[3]

Although the field of microbiome research is amazing and has uncovered fascinating things happening right under our noses without us ever realizing it, some scientists are concerned that the field has been "more driven by methods than by hypotheses or concepts" (see note 2). The over-reliance on metagenomics is noticeable. This may stem from a widespread misconception that most microbes are unculturable but as we have seen, the rediscovery of traditional culture techniques and the exciting new field of "culturomics" have shown this to be false. There is a dawning recognition in the microbiome world that being able to lay our hands on an actual microbe, rather than just considering a computer-generated version of its genome, really is essential for further understanding of these microbes.[4]

As well as an overreliance on genetic techniques, we have also seen an overreliance on analyzing stool samples, that homogenous and somewhat uninformative summary of the gut. Perhaps in the future, there will start to be more of a focus on the microarchitecture of each biohabitat, as exemplified by the biopsies taken for the probiotic trial discussed in the probiotic chapter. Another important technique to rediscover is the 19th- and 20th-century skill of counting microbes (becoming more prevalent with the use of flow cytometry), and now that metagenomic techniques are reducing in cost, an effort to take samples more frequently. Flow cytometry would give an idea of a microbe's prevalence and more frequent samples a sense of the temporal change within a microbiome, both aspects giving more context, more information on a microbe's relevance. Like old-fashioned Victorian archaeology, when gold artifacts were dug up without recording the context of the finds, digging up lists of microbes in the gut has little value on its own. Without knowledge of the context in which these microbes are found, microbiome research becomes merely a sequence of stamp collecting, a collecting of the infinite varieties of microbial species found in the gut, without considering the import of the microbes present (if any).[5]

Microbiome research, of course, overlaps with many other well-established scientific specialties to the benefit of both, and in particular a fertile partnership with geneticists and evolutionary specialists has developed. Discussions comparing microbiomes between different animals and the microbial coevolution that this implies are some of the most interesting and informative in the microbiome field.

210 THE MICROBIOME

There are, of course, some inaccurate assumptions prevalent in microbiome research that need further attention. The assumption that we live in a microbial world and that the biology of all animals is mediated by microbiomes is not correct. A microbiome is not inescapable. As we have touched on very briefly (and would have loved to focus more on), not all animals have or need a microbiome. Some animals have invested in excluding microbes completely by living in the sterile tissues of another animal, and others by simply not utilizing their effects in the digestive tracts, even when they tolerate their presence (see note 3). Another assumption—that microorganisms are either beneficial, pathogenic, or neutral according to microbial interactions with their hosts—is based on an anthropocentric view and also not quite right (see note 2). There are also difficulties in using loaded or political words such as "communities" and "diversity" with respect to the microbiome, which can lead to misinterpretations even among scientists, as they pick up on the political zeitgeist of our time.

The major problematic idea gaining traction is that we, as humans plus microbes, are somehow "superorganisms." The concept of superorganisms, "a view gaining in popularity," is the idea that a human and its microbiome are a unit of evolutionary selection and that, therefore, this unit has properties similar to an individual organism. This implies that we have evolved into some sort of super-energized and creative creature. The problem with this view (one of the many problems) is that it assumes that every interaction between us and our microbes is a positive one. This means many research papers—indeed the whole flavor of microbiome research—appear only concerned "with cooperative and integrative features . . . to the exclusion of other kinds of interactions," ignoring any competition between microorganisms and any conflicts between hosts and microbial "partners." Simply put, entire microbiomes do not evolve as single units with their hosts. We are not superorganisms.[6]

However, as we have seen, we do live together, we do interact, and we do benefit somewhat from the interactions we have with microbes—although we can survive without them. More prosaic but unfortunately less beautiful is the likelihood that each of us is simply living off the waste products of the other. If microbes "perform a useful function, even if just through a by-product of microbial metabolism, a host may evolve mechanisms to favour these bacterial species and thereby reinforce their effects."[7] And as we have seen, even when the effects of microbes are not beneficial, we may still become dependent on their presence.

The promotion of ideas such as "superorganisms" or claims that knowledge of the microbiome "is beginning to call into question what it means to be human" are typical examples of the overhyping and overselling of microbiome research that goes on. Embarrassingly, this is easily debunked, even by nonspecialists, who point out "most of these claims are made in a single sentence without further development or defence, often as a catchy opening line."[8] The microbiome is fascinating as it is. It doesn't need this hype.

The endless variability of the human microbiome is easily one of the biggest challenges to interpret. It is likely, though, that this just reflects the endless variety of microbes in the environment. As Escherich observed right back in 1884, the variability of the microbes in our gut is "a situation that seems controlled by a thousand coincidences." Although we are desperate to apply the lessons learned in microbiome research to medical practice, "understanding what proportion of this variance is medically important and clinically actionable" is exceptionally difficult. A very small proportion perhaps, mainly relating to that slight effect the microbiome has on our calorie absorption, the slight effect it has on protecting our babies from pathogens, and the observations we have made concerning the development of allergies.[9]

A diverse microbiome is at least widely regarded to be a healthy microbiome, especially when it comes to our gut. But does diversity in our microbiomes actually matter with respect to developing allergies? A diverse skin or gut microbiome is a natural result of exposure to the environment but could be argued as not necessarily healthy or useful in itself. Although our rates of allergy—especially in children—are clearly reduced by constant exposure to microbes, this might not be the result of having a diverse microbiome, which may in the end merely be a surrogate measure for assessing rates of microbial exposure.

212 THE MICROBIOME

So, is anything we have discovered directly useful to us right now? Where is the translational impact?

It may be that having read this book we will be motivated to ditch shower gel and enable the protective barriers of our skin to work more effectively. Or that we decide to eat a wider variety of whole foods and, in particular, more fiber in order to preserve the innate immune barrier systems within our gut, our mucus. We may also be able to save a few dollars if we are inclined not to bother with conventional probiotics anymore. Perhaps we will continue to particularly enjoy fermented foods—not because they are especially healthy but just for the fun of knowing we are eating millions of microbes at one time. We now know that if we are healthy and if our immune system and barrier systems are working normally, we can cope perfectly well with these kinds of foods, as many of us do the world over as part of a natural diet. And if we can all get out of our homes more and enjoy natural spaces and plants, contact with soil, animals, and each other, then all the better. There are many good reasons to get out of the house: for company, for sunlight, for exercise, and for good mental health.

The key health messages from the World Health Organization are still correct. We don't need any knowledge of the microbiome to develop these or to adjust them. For all of the things we have talked about; childbirth, breastfeeding, standard aseptic procedures, hand decontamination, food preparation, drinking water safety, safe sex, and everything else, the guidance is already in place.

It may be that the era of live biotherapeutics is just around the corner with regard to *Clostridium difficile* and *Lactobacillus crispii*, but we can note that these are specific microbes toted for specific pathogens, not some kind of community effort of microbes bringing back balance to our lives.

And lastly, we don't ever want to forget the lessons of germ theory, the death rates in our cities of one in thirty citizens per year, or the epidemics of the 19th century. We want to keep on with ordinary handwashing, food hygiene, sewage disposal, clean water, and ordinary preventive medical care and live an ordinary and healthy life.

Be confident. We are mainly doing everything right.

NOTES

Chapter 1

1. Whipps, J. M., J. A. Lewis, and R. J. Cook. "Mycoparasitism and Plant Control." In *Fungi in Biological Control Systems*, edited by M. N. Burge, 176. Manchester: Manchester University Press, 1988.

2. Berg, Gabriele, Daria Rybakova, Dominik Fischer, et al. "Microbiome Definition Re-Visited: Old Concepts and New Challenges." *Microbiome* 8 (2020): 103. https://doi.org/10.1186/s40168-020-00875-0.

3. Sender, Ron, Shai Fuchs, and Ron Milo. "Revised Estimates for the Number of Human and Bacteria Cells in the Body." *PLOS Biology* 14, no. 8 (2016): e1002533. https://doi.org/10.1371/journal.pbio.1002533.

4. Chalifour, B. N., L. E. Elder, and J. Li. "Gut Microbiome of Century-Old Snail Specimens Stable across Time in Preservation." *Microbiome* 10 (2022): 99. https://doi.org/10.1186/s40168-022-01286-z.

5. Andrewes, F. W. "The Nomenclature and Classification of Micro-Organisms." In *A System of Bacteriology in Relation to Medicine*, Vol. 1, 60. London: Medical Research Council, 1930.

6. Leidy, Joseph. "Morphology of the Bacteria (Vibrio and Spirillum), an Early Research.—The Intestinal Flora." *Science*, New Series, 40, no. 1026 (August 28, 1914): 302–306. https://www.jstor.org/stable/1640989.

7. Littman, R. J. "The Plague of Athens: Epidemiology and Paleopathology." *Mount Sinai Journal of Medicine* 76, no. 5 (2009): 456–467. https://doi.org/10.1002/msj.20137.

8. Chadwick, Edwin. *Report on the Sanitary Condition of the Labouring Population and on the Means of Its Improvement*. London: W. Clowes and Sons, 1842.

9. Shattuck, Lemuel. *Report of a General Plan for the promotion of general and public health devised, prepared and recommended by the commissioners appointed under a resolve of the legislature of Massachusetts, relating to a sanitary survey of the state*. Boston: Dutton and Wentworth State Printers, 1850.

10. Woodham-Smith, Cecil. *Florence Nightingale*. London: Constable and Company Ltd, 1950.

11. Bulloch, William. "The History of Bacteriology." In *A System of Bacteriology in Relation to Medicine*, Vol. 1, 60. London: Medical Research Council, 1930.

214 NOTES

12. Ducleux, Emile. *A History of a Mind.* Philadelphia and London: W. B. Saunders Company, 1920.
13. Morrey, Charles Bradfield. *The Fundamentals of Bacteriology.* New York: Lea and Febiger, 1921.

Chapter 2

1. *The W. Heath Robinson Illustrated Story Book.* London: The Hamlyn Publishing Group Limited, 1979.
2. Darwin, Charles. "An Account of the Fine Dust Which Often Falls on Vessels in the Atlantic Ocean." *Quarterly Journal of the Geological Society* 2 (1846): 26–30. https://doi.org/10.1144/GSL.JGS.1846.002.01-02.09.
3. Reche, Isabel, Gianluca D'Orta, Nikolay Mladenov, Dana M. Winget, and Curtis A. Suttle. "Deposition Rates of Viruses and Bacteria above the Atmospheric Boundary Layer." *ISME Journal* 12, no. 4 (2018): 1154–1162. https://doi.org/10.1038/s41396-017-0042-4.
4. Ashuro, Z., K. Diriba, A. Afework, G. Husen Washo, A. Shiferaw Areba, G. G/Meskel Kanno, H. E. Hareru, A. W. Kaso, and M. Tesfu. "Assessment of Microbiological Quality of Indoor Air at Different Hospital Sites of Dilla University: A Cross-Sectional Study." *Environmental Health Insights* 16 (2022): 11786302221100047. https://doi.org/10.1177/11786302221100047.
5. Banerjee, S., and M. G. A. van der Heijden. "Soil Microbiomes and One Health." *Nature Reviews Microbiology* 21 (2023): 6–20. https://doi.org/10.1038/s41579-022-00779.
6. Wallace, T. C., F. Guarner, K. Madsen, M. D. Cabana, G. Gibson, E. Hentges, and M. E. Sanders. "Human Gut Microbiota and Its Relationship to Health and Disease." *Nutrition Reviews* 69, no. 7 (2011): 392–403. https://doi.org/10.1111/j.1753-4887.2011.00402.x.
7. Gordon, H. A., and L. Pesti. "The Gnotobiotic Animal as a Tool in the Study of Host Microbial Relationships." *Bacteriological Reviews* 35, no. 4 (1971): 390–429.
8. Reyniers, J. A. "Germ-Free Vertebrates: Present Status." *Annals of the New York Academy of Sciences* 78 (1959): 1–400.
9. Williams, S. C. P. "Gnotobiotics." *PNAS* 111, no. 5 (February 4, 2014): 1661.
10. Scott, Katie Collins. "Former University of Portland President Listed in Grand Jury Abuse Report." *National Catholic Reporter*, September 25, 2018.
11. Lawrence, R. J., and M. A. Murphy. *Bursting the Bubble: The Tortured Life and Untimely Death of David Vetter.* Augustine Moore Press, 2019.
12. Williamson, A., J. Montgomery, M. South, et al. "A Special Report: Four-Year Study of a Boy with Combined Immune Deficiency Maintained in Strict Reverse Isolation from Birth." *Pediatric Research* 11 (1977): 63–64. https://doi.org/10.1203/00006450-197701000-00001.
13. Fuhrman, J. A., K. McCallum, and A. A. Davis. "Novel Major Archaebacterial Group from Marine Plankton." *Nature* 356, no. 6365 (1992): 148–149. https://doi.org/10.1038/356148a0.

14. DeLong, E. F. "Archaea in Coastal Marine Environments." *Proceedings of the National Academy of Sciences* 89, no. 12 (1992): https://doi.org/10.1073/pnas.89.12.5685.
15. Woese, C. R., and G. E. Fox. "Phylogenetic Structure of the Prokaryotic Domain: The Primary Kingdoms." *Proceedings of the National Academy of Sciences* 74, no. 11 (1977): 5088–5090. https://doi.org/10.1073/pnas.74.11.5088. "We thank Linda Madrum and David Nanney for suggesting the name 'archaebacteria.'"
16. Pace, Norman. "Time for a Change." *Nature* 441 (2006): 289.
17. Venter, J. C., K. Remington, J. F. Heidelberg, et al. "Environmental Genome Shotgun Sequencing of the Sargasso Sea." *Science* 304, no. 5667 (2004): 66–74. https://doi.org/10.1126/science.1093857.
18. Baveye, Philippe C. "Bypass and Hyperbole in Soil Research: Worrisome Practices Critically Reviewed through Examples." *European Journal of Soil Science* 72 (2021): 1–20.
19. National Research Council. *The New Science of Metagenomics: Revealing the Secrets of Our Microbial Planet.* Washington, DC: National Academies Press, 2007.
20. Turnbaugh, P. J., R. E. Ley, M. Hamady, et al. "The Human Microbiome Project." *Nature* 449, no. 7164 (2007): 804–810. https://doi.org/10.1038/nature06244.
21. Proctor, L. M. "The Human Microbiome Project in 2011 and Beyond." *Cell Host & Microbe* 10, no. 4 (2011): 287–291. https://doi.org/10.1016/j.chom.2011.10.001.
22. Proctor, L. M. "Priorities for the Next 10 Years of Human Microbiome Research." *Nature* 569 (2019): 623–625.
23. NIH Human Microbiome Portfolio Analysis Team. "A Review of 10 Years of Human Microbiome Research Activities at the US National Institutes of Health, Fiscal Years 2007–2016." *Microbiome* 7, no. 1 (2019): 31. https://doi.org/10.1186/s40168-019-0620-y.

Chapter 3

1. Montes, Leopoldo F., and Walter H. Wilborn. "Location of Bacterial Skin Flora." *British Journal of Dermatology* 81, no. s1 (January 1, 1969): 23–26. https://doi.org/10.1111/j.1365-2133.1969.tb12829.x.
2. Smith, F. W., and M. Bruch. "Reduction of Microbiological Shedding in Clean Rooms." *Developments in Industrial Microbiology* 10 (1969): 290.
3. Leung, Marcus H. Y., David Wilkins, Ellen K. T. Li, Fred K. F. Kong, and Patrick K. H. Lee. "Indoor-Air Microbiome in an Urban Subway Network: Diversity and Dynamics." ORCID: http://orcid.org/0000-0002-6342-8181.
4. Price, Philip B. "The Bacteriology of Normal Skin1." *The Journal of Infectious Diseases* 63, no. 3 (November–December 1938): 301–318. Oxford University Press.
5. Welch. *General Bacteriology of Surgical Infections.* Vol. 1, p. 250. Philadelphia, 1895.
6. Edmonds-Wilson, S. L., N. I. Nurinova, C. A. Zapka, N. Fierer, and M. Wilson. "Review of Human Hand Microbiome Research." *Journal of Dermatological Science* 80, no. 1 (October 2015): 3–12. https://doi.org/10.1016/j.jdermsci.2015.07.006.
7. Byrd, A., Y. Belkaid, and J. Segre. "The Human Skin Microbiome." *Nature Reviews Microbiology* 16 (2018): 143–155. https://doi.org/10.1038/nrmicro.2017.157.

216 NOTES

8. Moissl-Eichinger, C., A. J. Probst, G. Birarda, et al. "Human Age and Skin Physiology Shape Diversity and Abundance of Archaea on Skin." *Scientific Reports* 7 (2017): 4039. https://doi.org/10.1038/s41598-017-04197-4.

9. Gillespie, J. J., A. R. Wattam, S. A. Cammer, et al. "PATRIC: The Comprehensive Bacterial Bioinformatics Resource with a Focus on Human Pathogenic Species." *Infection and Immunity* 79, no. 11 (2011): 4286–4298. https://doi.org/10.1128/IAI. 00207-11.

10. Sollid, J. U. E., A. S. Furberg, A. M. Hanssen, and M. Johannessen. "Staphylococcus aureus: Determinants of Human Carriage." *Infection, Genetics and Evolution* 21 (2014): 531–541.

11. Evans, C. A., W. M. Smith, E. A. Johnston, and E. R. Giblett. "Bacterial Flora of the Normal Human Skin." *Journal of Investigative Dermatology* 15, no. 4 (October 1950): 305–324. https://doi.org/10.1038/jid.1950.105.

12. Severn, M. M., and A. R. Horswill. "Staphylococcus epidermidis and Its Dual Lifestyle in Skin Health and Infection." *Nature Reviews Microbiology* 21 (2023): 97–111. https://doi.org/10.1038/s41579-022-00780-3.

13. Edmonds-Wilson, S. L., N. I. Nurinova, C. A. Zapka, N. Fierer, and M. Wilson. "Review of Human Hand Microbiome Research." *Journal of Dermatological Science* 80, no. 1 (October 2015): 3–12. https://doi.org/10.1016/j.jdermsci.2015.07.006.

14. Lax, Simon. "Longitudinal Analysis of Microbial Interaction between Humans and the Indoor Environment." *Science* 345, no. 6200 (August 29, 2014): 1048–1052. https://doi.org/10.1126/science.1254529.

15. Zhang, N., W. Jia, P. Wang, et al. "Most Self-Touches Are with the Nondominant Hand." *Scientific Reports* 10 (2020): 10457. https://doi.org/10.1038/s41598-020-67521-5.

16. Fierer, Noah. "The Influence of Sex, Handedness, and Washing on the Diversity of Hand Surface Bacteria." *Proceedings of the National Academy of Sciences* 105, no. 46 (November 18, 2008): 17994–17999. https://doi.org/10.1073/pnas. 0807920105.

17. Wilkins, D., X. Tong, M. H. Y. Leung, et al. "Diurnal Variation in the Human Skin Microbiome Affects Accuracy of Forensic Microbiome Matching." *Microbiome* 9 (2021): 129. https://doi.org/10.1186/s40168-021-01082-1.

18. World Health Organization. *WHO Guidelines on Hand Hygiene in Health Care.* Geneva: WHO, 2009.

19. Skinner, F. A. *The Normal Microbial Flora of Man.* London: Academic Press, 1974, p. 17.

20. Larson, Elaine. "Skin Hygiene and Infection Prevention: More of the Same or Different Approaches?" *Clinical Infectious Diseases* 29, no. 5 (November 1999): 1287–1294. https://doi.org/10.1086/313468.

21. Rosenthal, M., A. Aiello, E. Larson, C. Chenoweth, and B. Foxman. "Healthcare Workers' Hand Microbiome May Mediate Carriage of Hospital Pathogens." *Pathogens* 3, no. 1 (December 27, 2013): 1–13. https://doi.org/10.3390/ pathogens3010001.

22. Gormley, N. J., A. C. Bronstein, J. J. Rasimas, et al. "The Rising Incidence of Intentional Ingestion of Ethanol-Containing Hand Sanitizers." *Critical Care Medicine*

40, no. 1 (January 2012): 290–294. https://doi.org/10.1097/CCM. 0b013e31822f09c0.

23. https://psnet.ahrq.gov/web-mm/hidden-harms-hand-sanitizer.

24. Zapka, C. A., E. J. Campbell, S. L. Maxwell, et al. "Bacterial Hand Contamination and Transfer after Use of Contaminated Bulk-Soap-Refillable Dispensers." *Applied and Environmental Microbiology* 77, no. 9 (May 2011): 2898–2904. https://doi.org/10.1128/AEM.02632-10.

25. Marples, R. R. "Effects of Soaps, Germicides and Disinfectants on Skin Flora." In *The Normal Microbial Flora of Man*, edited by F. A. Skinner. London and New York: Academic Press, 1974.

26. Jamieson, W. Allan. "An Address Delivered at the Opening of the Section of Dermatology." *BMJ*, August 26, 1893, 455.

27. Stowers, J. H. "Bacteria in Diseases of the Skin." *Transactions of the Dermatology Society of Great Britain and Ireland* 3 (1897): 14.

28. George, S. M. C., S. Karanovic, D. A. Harrison, et al. "Interventions to Reduce Staphylococcus aureus in the Management of Eczema." *Cochrane Database of Systematic Reviews* 2019, no. 10: CD003871. https://doi.org/10.1002/14651858. CD003871.pub3.

Chapter 4

1. Escherich, T. "The Intestinal Bacteria of the Neonate and Breast-Fed Infant. 1884." *Reviews of Infectious Diseases* 10, no. 6 (November–December 1988): 1220–25. https://doi.org/10.1093/clinids/10.6.1220.

2. Steckel, Richard H., and Roderick Floud, eds. *Health and Welfare during Industrialization*. Chicago: University of Chicago Press, 1997. http://www.nber.org/books/stec97-1.

3. Twarog, Sophia. "Heights and Living Standards in Germany, 1850–1939: The Case of Wurttemberg." In *Health and Welfare during Industrialization*, 285–330. http://www.nber.org/chapters/c7434.

4. Cruickshank, Robert. "Bacillus Bifidus: Its Characters and Isolation from the Intestine of Infants." *The Journal of Hygiene* 24, no. 3/4 (1925): 241–54. http://www.jstor.org/stable/3859532.

5. Friedmann, Herbert C. "Escherich and Escherichia." In *Advances in Applied Microbiology*, vol. 60, 160. 2006.

6. Hall, R. T., and O'Toole, J. "Bacterial Flora of First Specimens of Meconium Passed by Fifty New-Born Infants." Denver, 1929.

7. Fanaro, S., R. Chierici, P. Guerrini, and V. Vigi. "Intestinal Microflora in Early Infancy: Composition and Development." *Acta Paediatrica Supplement* 91, no. 441 (September 2003): 48–55. https://doi.org/10.1111/j.1651-2227.2003.tb00646.x.

8. Ferretti, P., et al. "Mother-to-Infant Microbial Transmission from Different Body Sites Shapes the Developing Infant Gut Microbiome." *Cell Host & Microbe* 24, no. 1 (July 11, 2018): 133–145.e5. https://doi.org/10.1016/j.chom.2018.06.005.

218 NOTES

9. Shin, H., Z. Pei, K. A. Martinez, et al. "The First Microbial Environment of Infants Born by C-Section: The Operating Room Microbes." *Microbiome* 3 (2015): 59. https://doi.org/10.1186/s40168-015-0126-1.

10. Sandall, J., et al. "Long-Term Risks and Benefits Associated with Caesarean Delivery for Mother, Baby and Subsequent Pregnancies: Systematic Review and Meta-Analysis." *PLOS Medicine* (January 23, 2018). https://doi.org/10.1371/journal.pmed.1002494.

11. Chu, D., J. Ma, A. Prince, et al. "Maturation of the Infant Microbiome Community Structure and Function across Multiple Body Sites and in Relation to Mode of Delivery." *Nature Medicine* 23 (2017): 314–326. https://doi.org/10.1038/nm.4272.

12. Aagaard, K., J. Ma, K. M. Antony, R. Ganu, J. Petrosino, and J. Versalovic. "The Placenta Harbors a Unique Microbiome." *Science Translational Medicine* 6, no. 237 (May 21, 2014): 237ra65. https://doi.org/10.1126/scitranslmed.3008599.

13. Nyangahu, D. D., and H. B. Jaspan. "Influence of Maternal Microbiota during Pregnancy on Infant Immunity." *Clinical and Experimental Immunology* 198, no. 1 (October 2019): 47–56. https://doi.org/10.1111/cei.13331.

14. Walter, J., and M. W. Hornef. "A Philosophical Perspective on the Prenatal In Utero Microbiome Debate." *Microbiome* 9 (2021): 5. https://doi.org/10.1186/s40168-020-00979-7.

15. Kennedy, K. M., M. J. Gerlach, T. Adam, et al. "Fetal Meconium Does Not Have a Detectable Microbiota before Birth." *Nature Microbiology* 6 (2021): 865–873. https://doi.org/10.1038/s41564-021-00904-0.

16. Kennedy, Katherine M., Marcus C. de Goffau, Maria Elisa Perez-Muñoz, Marie-Claire Arrieta, Fredrik Bäckhed, Peer Bork, Thorsten Braun, et al. *"Questioning the Fetal Microbiome Illustrates Pitfalls of Low-Biomass Microbial Studies."* *Nature* 613, no. 7945 (January 2023): 639–649. https://doi.org/10.1038/s41586-022-05546-8.

17. Bartlett, A., D. Padfield, L. Lear, R. Bendall, and M. Vos. "A Comprehensive List of Bacterial Pathogens Infecting Humans." *Microbiology (Reading)* 168, no. 12 (December 2022). https://doi.org/10.1099/mic.0.001269.

18. Adlerberth, I., and A. E. Wold. "Establishment of the Gut Microbiota in Western Infants." *Acta Paediatrica* 98, no. 2 (February 2009): 229–238. https://doi.org/10.1111/j.1651-2227.2008.01060.x.

19. Karabayır, Nalan, Tülin A. Özden, Özlem Durmaz, and Gülbin Gökçay. "Fecal Calprotectin Levels in the Babies with Infantile Colic." *Journal of Child* 21, no. 2 (2021): 105–110. https://doi.org/10.26650/jchild.2021.775736.

20. Rhoads, J. M., J. Collins, N. Y. Fatheree, et al. "Infant Colic Represents Gut Inflammation and Dysbiosis." *Journal of Pediatrics* 203 (December 2018): 55–61.e3. https://doi.org/10.1016/j.jpeds.2018.07.042.

21. Turroni, F., C. Milani, S. Duranti, et al. "Bifidobacteria and the Infant Gut: An Example of Co-Evolution and Natural Selection." *Cellular and Molecular Life Sciences* 75 (2018): 103–118. https://doi.org/10.1007/s00018-017-2672-0.

22. Cruickshank, R. "Bacillus Bifidus: Its Characters and Isolation from the Intestine of Infants." *Journal of Hygiene* 24, no. 3–4 (1925): 241–254. https://doi.org/10.1017/S0022172400008718.

Notes 219

23. Rettger, L. F. "The Influence of Milk Feeding on Mortality and Growth, and on the Character of the Intestinal Flora." *Journal of Experimental Medicine* 21, no. 4 (April 1, 1915): 365–388. https://doi.org/10.1084/jem.21.4.365.

24. Dalby, M. J., and L. J. Hall. "Recent Advances in Understanding the Neonatal Microbiome." *F1000Research* 9 (May 22, 2020): F1000 Faculty Rev-422. https://doi.org/10.12688/f1000research.22355.1.

25. Lawson, M. A. E., I. J. O'Neill, M. Kujawska, et al. "Breast Milk-Derived Human Milk Oligosaccharides Promote Bifidobacterium Interactions within a Single Ecosystem." *ISME Journal* 14 (2020): 635–648. https://doi.org/10.1038/s41396-019-0553-2.

26. O'Callaghan, A., and D. van Sinderen. "Bifidobacteria and Their Role as Members of the Human Gut Microbiota." *Frontiers in Microbiology* 7 (June 15, 2016): 925. https://doi.org/10.3389/fmicb.2016.00925.

27. Wiciński, M., E. Sawicka, J. Gębalski, K. Kubiak, and B. Malinowski. "Human Milk Oligosaccharides: Health Benefits, Potential Applications in Infant Formulas, and Pharmacology." *Nutrients* 12, no. 1 (January 20, 2020): 266. https://doi.org/10.3390/nu12010266.

28. Tannock, G. W., P. S. Lee, K. H. Wong, and B. Lawley. "Why Don't All Infants Have Bifidobacteria in Their Stool?" *Frontiers in Microbiology* 7 (May 31, 2016): 834. https://doi.org/10.3389/fmicb.2016.00834.

29. Kramer, M. S., B. Chalmers, E. D. Hodnett, et al. "Promotion of Breastfeeding Intervention Trial (PROBIT): A Randomized Trial in the Republic of Belarus." *JAMA* 285, no. 4 (January 24–31, 2001): 413–420. https://doi.org/10.1001/jama.285.4.413.

Chapter 5

1. Rogers, A. P., S. J. Mileto, and D. Lyras. "Impact of Enteric Bacterial Infections at and beyond the Epithelial Barrier." *Nature Reviews Microbiology* 21 (2023): 260–274. https://doi.org/10.1038/s41579-022-00794-x.

2. Hammer, Tobin J., et al. "Not All Animals Need a Microbiome." *FEMS Microbiology Letters* 366, no. 10 (May 2019): fnz117. https://doi.org/10.1093/femsle/fnz117.

3. Wilson, Michael. *The Human Microbiota in Health and Disease.* Boca Raton: CRC Press, 2019, 361.

4. Rajilić-Stojanović, M., and W. M. de Vos. "The First 1000 Cultured Species of the Human Gastrointestinal Microbiota." *FEMS Microbiology Reviews* 38, no. 5 (September 2014): 996–1047. https://doi.org/10.1111/1574-6976.12075.

5. Turnbaugh, P. J., R. E. Ley, M. A. Mahowald, V. Magrini, E. R. Mardis, and J. I. Gordon. "An Obesity-Associated Gut Microbiome with Increased Capacity for Energy Harvest." *Nature* 444, no. 7122 (December 21, 2006): 1027–1031. https://doi.org/10.1038/nature05414.

6. Eckburg, P. B., E. M. Bik, C. N. Bernstein, et al. "Diversity of the Human Intestinal Microbial Flora." *Science* 308, no. 5728 (June 10, 2005): 1635–1638. https://doi.org/10.1126/science.1110591.

7. Qin, J., et al. "A Human Gut Microbial Gene Catalogue Established by Metagenomic Sequencing." *Nature* 464 (2010): 59–65. https://doi.org/10.1038/nature08821.

220 NOTES

8. Chibani, C. M., A. Mahnert, G. Borrel, et al. "A Catalogue of 1,167 Genomes from the Human Gut Archaeome." *Nature Microbiology* 7, no. 1 (January 2022): 48–61. https://doi.org/10.1038/s41564-021-01020-9. Erratum in: *Nature Microbiology* 7, no. 2 (2022): 339. https://doi.org/10.1038/s41564-022-01039-9.

9. Zuppi, M., H. L. Hendrickson, J. M. O'Sullivan, and T. Vatanen. "Phages in the Gut Ecosystem." *Frontiers in Cellular and Infection Microbiology* 11 (2022): 822562. https://doi.org/10.3389/fcimb.2021.822562.

10. Alarcón-Schumacher, T., and S. Erdmann. "A Trove of Asgard Archaeal Viruses." *Nature Microbiology* 7 (2022): 931–932. https://doi.org/10.1038/s41564-022-01148-2.

11. Hedlund, B. P., M. Chuvochina, P. Hugenholtz, et al. "SeqCode: A Nomenclatural Code for Prokaryotes Described from Sequence Data." *Nature Microbiology* 7 (2022): 1702–1708. https://doi.org/10.1038/s41564-022-01214-9.

12. Sergaki, C., S. Anwar, M. Fritzsche, et al. "Developing Whole Cell Standards for the Microbiome Field." *Microbiome* 10 (2022): 123. https://doi.org/10.1186/s40168-022-01313-z.

13. https://www.nibsc.org/products/brm_product_catalogue/detail_page.aspx?catid=20/302.

14. Lagier, J. C., G. Dubourg, M. Million, et al. "Culturing the Human Microbiota and Culturomics." *Nature Reviews Microbiology* 16 (2018): 540–550. https://doi.org/10.1038/s41579-018-0041-0.

15. Seng, P., M. Drancourt, F. Gouriet, et al. "Ongoing Revolution in Bacteriology: Routine Identification of Bacteria by Matrix-Assisted Laser Desorption Ionization Time-of-Flight Mass Spectrometry." *Clinical Infectious Diseases* 49, no. 4 (August 15, 2009): 543–551. https://doi.org/10.1086/600885.

16. Lagier, J. C., F. Armougom, M. Million, et al. "Microbial Culturomics: Paradigm Shift in the Human Gut Microbiome Study." *Clinical Microbiology and Infection* 18, no. 12 (December 2012): 1185–1193. https://doi.org/10.1111/1469-0691.12023.

17. Hammer, Tobin J., Jon G. Sanders, and Noah Fierer. "Not All Animals Need a Microbiome." *FEMS Microbiology Letters* 366, no. 10 (May 2019): fnz117. https://doi.org/10.1093/femsle/fnz117.

18. Derrien, M., and J. E. van Hylckama Vlieg. "Fate, Activity, and Impact of Ingested Bacteria within the Human Gut Microbiota." *Trends in Microbiology* 23, no. 6 (June 2015): 354–366. https://doi.org/10.1016/j.tim.2015.03.002.

19. Leff, J. W., and N. Fierer. "Bacterial Communities Associated with the Surfaces of Fresh Fruits and Vegetables." *PLoS ONE* 8, no. 3 (2013): e59310. https://doi.org/10.1371/journal.pone.0059310.

20. Lang, J. M., J. A. Eisen, and A. M. Zivkovic. "The Microbes We Eat: Abundance and Taxonomy of Microbes Consumed in a Day's Worth of Meals for Three Diet Types." *PeerJ* 2 (2014): e659. https://doi.org/10.7717/peerj.659.

21. Derrien, M., and J. E. van Hylckama Vlieg. "Fate, Activity, and Impact of Ingested Bacteria within the Human Gut Microbiota." *Trends in Microbiology* 23, no. 6 (June 2015): 354–366. https://doi.org/10.1016/j.tim.2015.03.002.

22. David, L., C. Maurice, R. Carmody, et al. "Diet Rapidly and Reproducibly Alters the Human Gut Microbiome." *Nature* 505 (2014): 559–563. https://doi.org/10.1038/nature12820.

Notes 221

23. Lesaulnier, C. C., C. W. Herbold, C. Pelikan, et al. "Bottled Aqua Incognita: Microbiota Assembly and Dissolved Organic Matter Diversity in Natural Mineral Waters." *Microbiome* 5 (2017): 126. https://doi.org/10.1186/s40168-017-0344-9.

24. Bartram, J., J., Cotruvo, M. Exner, C. Fricker, and A. Glasmacher, eds. *Heterotrophic Plate Counts and Drinking-Water Safety: The Significance of HPCs for Water Quality and Human Health.* Geneva: World Health Organization, 2003.

25. Barker, J., and M. V. Jones. "The Potential Spread of Infection Caused by Aerosol Contamination of Surfaces after Flushing a Domestic Toilet." *Journal of Applied Microbiology* 99, no. 2 (2005): 339–347. https://doi.org/10.1111/j.1365-2672.2005.02610.x.

26. Gacesa, R., A. Kurilshikov, A. Vich Vila, et al. "Environmental Factors Shaping the Gut Microbiome in a Dutch Population." *Nature* 604 (2022): 732–739. https://doi.org/10.1038/s41586-022-04567-1.

27. King, C. H. "Baseline Human Gut Microbiota Profile in Healthy People and Standard Reporting Template." *PLoS ONE* 14, no. 9 (September 11, 2019): e0206484. https://doi.org/10.1371/journal.pone.0206484.

28. Risely, Alice. "Applying the Core Microbiome to Understand Host–Microbe Systems." *Journal of Animal Ecology* 89, no. 7 (2020): 1549–1558.

29. Wostmann, B. S., C. Larkin, A. Moriarty, and E. Bruckner-Kardoss. "Dietary Intake, Energy Metabolism, and Excretory Losses of Adult Male Germfree Wistar Rats." *Laboratory Animal Science* 33, no. 1 (February 1983): 46–50.

30. Wostmann, Bernard S. *Germ Free and Gnotobiotic Animals.* Notre Dame, IN: CRC Press, 1996.

31. Mortimer, Ian. *Medieval Horizons: Why the Middle Ages Matter.* London: Bodley Head, 2023.

32. Sanders, Jon G., Piotr Łukasik, Megan E. Frederickson, et al. "Dramatic Differences in Gut Bacterial Densities Correlate with Diet and Habitat in Rainforest Ants." *Integrative and Comparative Biology* 57, no. 4 (October 2017): 705–722. https://doi.org/10.1093/icb/icx088.

33. Gordon, H. A. "Is the Germ-Free Animal Normal?" In *The Germ-Free Animal in Research*, edited by Coates, Chapter 6. London: Academic Press, 1968.

34. Karl, J. Philip, et al. "Fecal Concentrations of Bacterially Derived Vitamin K Forms Are Associated with Gut Microbiota Composition but Not Plasma or Fecal Cytokine Concentrations in Healthy Adults." *The American Journal of Clinical Nutrition* 106, no. 4 (2017): 1052–1061.

35. Sonnenburg, E., S. Smits, M. Tikhonov, et al. "Diet-Induced Extinctions in the Gut Microbiota Compound over Generations." *Nature* 529 (2016): 212–215. https://doi.org/10.1038/nature16504.

36. Subramanian, S., S. Huq, T. Yatsunenko, et al. "Persistent Gut Microbiota Immaturity in Malnourished Bangladeshi Children." *Nature* 510 (2014): 417–421. https://doi.org/10.1038/nature13421.

37. Gehrig, Jeanette L., et al. "Effects of Microbiota-Directed Foods in Gnotobiotic Animals and Undernourished Children." *Science* 365 (2019): eaau4732. https://doi.org/10.1126/science.aau4732.

222 NOTES

38. Johansson, M. E., H. Sjövall, and G. C. Hansson. "The Gastrointestinal Mucus System in Health and Disease." *Nature Reviews Gastroenterology & Hepatology* 10, no. 6 (June 2013): 352–361. https://doi.org/10.1038/nrgastro.2013.35.
39. Bäckhed, Fredrik, et al. "Host-Bacterial Mutualism in the Human Intestine." *Science* 307 (2005): 1915–1920. https://doi.org/10.1126/science.1104816.
40. Bonfini, A., X. Liu, and N. Buchon. "From Pathogens to Microbiota: How Drosophila Intestinal Stem Cells React to Gut Microbes." *Developmental and Comparative Immunology* 64 (November 2016): 22–38. https://doi.org/10.1016/j.dci.2016.02.008.
41. Desai, Mahesh S., et al. "A Dietary Fiber-Deprived Gut Microbiota Degrades the Colonic Mucus Barrier and Enhances Pathogen Susceptibility." *Cell* 167, no. 5 (2016): 1339–1353. https://doi.org/10.1016/j.cell.2016.10.043.

Chapter 6

1. Mayer, Emeran A., Rob Knight, Sarkis K. Mazmanian, John F. Cryan, and Kirsten Tillisch. "Gut Microbes and the Brain: Paradigm Shift in Neuroscience." *Journal of Neuroscience* 34, no. 46 (November 12, 2014): 15490–96. https://doi.org/10.1523/JNEUROSCI.3299-14.2014.
2. Luczynski, Paulina, Karen A. McVey Neufeld, Ciara S. Oriach, Gerard Clarke, Timothy G. Dinan, and John F. Cryan. "Growing up in a Bubble: Using Germ-Free Animals to Assess the Influence of the Gut Microbiota on Brain and Behavior." *International Journal of Neuropsychopharmacology* 19, no. 8 (August 12, 2016): pyw020. https://doi.org/10.1093/ijnp/pyw020.
3. Dinan, Timothy G., and John F. Cryan. "Mood by Microbe: Towards Clinical Translation." *Genome Medicine* 8 (2016): 36. https://doi.org/10.1186/s13073-016-0292-1.
4. *Oxford Dictionary of Phrase and Fable.*
5. Miller, Ian. "The Gut-Brain Axis: Historical Reflections." *Microbial Ecology in Health and Disease* 29, no. 1 (November 8, 2018): 1542921. https://doi.org/10.1080/16512235.2018.1542921.
6. Koloski, Natasha A., Michael Jones, and Nicholas J. Talley. "Evidence That Independent Gut-to-Brain and Brain-to-Gut Pathways Operate in the Irritable Bowel Syndrome and Functional Dyspepsia: A 1-Year Population-Based Prospective Study." *Alimentary Pharmacology & Therapeutics* 44, no. 6 (September 2016): 592–600. https://doi.org/10.1111/apt.13738.
7. Mawe, Gary M., and James M. Hoffman. "Serotonin Signalling in the Gut—Functions, Dysfunctions and Therapeutic Targets." *Nature Reviews Gastroenterology & Hepatology* 10, no. 8 (August 2013): 473–86. https://doi.org/10.1038/nrgastro.2013.105.
8. Wostmann, Bernard S. *Germfree and Gnotobiotic Animals.* CRC Press, 1996.
9. Coates, M. E., ed. *The Germ-Free Animal in Research.* Academic Press, 1968.
10. Gordon, H. A. "Morphological and Physiological Characterization of Germfree Life." *Annals of the New York Academy of Sciences* 78 (May 8, 1959): 208–20. https://doi.org/10.1111/j.1749-6632.1959.tb53104.x.

Notes 223

11. Rader, Karen. *Making Mice: Standardising Mice for American Biomedical Research.* Princeton University Press, 2004.
12. Carbone, Larry. "Estimating Mouse and Rat Use in American Laboratories by Extrapolation from Animal Welfare Act-Regulated Species." *Scientific Reports* 11 (2021): 493. https://doi.org/10.1038/s41598-020-79961-0.
13. Neufeld, Karen M., Nancy Kang, John Bienenstock, and Jane A. Foster. "Reduced Anxiety-like Behavior and Central Neurochemical Change in Germ-Free Mice." *Neurogastroenterology & Motility* 23, no. 3 (March 2011): 255–64, e119. https://doi.org/10.1111/j.1365-2982.2010.01620.x.
14. Diaz Heijtz, Rochellys, Shan Wang, Faraz Anuar, et al. "Normal Gut Microbiota Modulates Brain Development and Behavior." *Proceedings of the National Academy of Sciences* 108, no. 7 (February 15, 2011): 3047–52. https://doi.org/10.1073/pnas.1010529108.
15. Bercik, Premysl, Emilie Denou, John Collins, et al. "The Intestinal Microbiota Affect Central Levels of Brain-Derived Neurotropic Factor and Behavior in Mice." *Gastroenterology* 141, no. 2 (August 2011): 599–609. https://doi.org/10.1053/j.gastro.2011.04.052.
16. https://phenome.jax.org/.
17. Crawley, Jacqueline. "Behavioural Phenotyping Strategies for Mutant Mice." *Neuron* 57 (2008): 809–18. https://doi.org/10.1016/j.neuron.2008.03.001.
18. Van Meer, Peter, and Jacob Raber. "Mouse Behavioural Analysis in Systems Biology." *Biochemical Journal* 389, no. Pt 3 (August 1, 2005): 593–610. https://doi.org/10.1042/BJ20042023.
19. Hooks, K. B., J. P. Konsman, and M. A. O'Malley. "Microbiota-Gut-Brain Research: A Critical Analysis." *Behavioral and Brain Sciences* 42 (2019): e60. https://doi.org/10.1017/S0140525X18002133.
20. Van Meer, Peter, and Jacob Raber. "Mouse Behavioural Analysis in Systems Biology." *Biochemical Journal* 389, no. Pt 3 (August 1, 2005): 593–610. https://doi.org/10.1042/BJ20042023.
21. Zimprich, Andreas, Lisa Garrett, Johannes M. Deussing, et al. "A Robust and Reliable Non-Invasive Test for Stress Responsivity in Mice." *Frontiers in Behavioral Neuroscience* 8 (April 15, 2014): 125. https://doi.org/10.3389/fnbeh.2014.00125.
22. Nguyen, T. L., S. Vieira-Silva, A. Liston, and J. Raes. "How Informative Is the Mouse for Human Gut Microbiota Research?" *Disease Models & Mechanisms* 8, no. 1 (January 2015): 1–16. https://doi.org/10.1242/dmm.017400.
23. Dinan, Timothy G., and John F. Cryan. "Mood by Microbe: Towards Clinical Translation." *Genome Medicine* 8 (2016): 36. https://doi.org/10.1186/s13073-016-0292-1.
24. Friedrich, M. J. "Unraveling the Influence of Gut Microbes on the Mind." *JAMA* 313, no. 17 (2015): 1699–1701. https://doi.org/10.1001/jama.2015.2159.
25. Nishino, R., K. Mikami, H. Takahashi, et al. "Commensal Microbiota Modulate Murine Behaviors in a Strictly Contamination-Free Environment Confirmed by Culture-Based Methods." *Neurogastroenterology & Motility* 25, no. 6 (June 2013): 521–528. https://doi.org/10.1111/nmo.12110.
26. https://mimedb.org/.

224 NOTES

27. Bérdy, J. "Bioactive Microbial Metabolites." *Journal of Antibiotics* 58 (2005): 1–26. https://doi.org/10.1038/ja.2005.1.

28. Silva, Y. P., A. Bernardi, and R. L. Frozza. "The Role of Short-Chain Fatty Acids from Gut Microbiota in Gut-Brain Communication." *Frontiers in Endocrinology* 11 (January 31, 2020): 25. https://doi.org/10.3389/fendo.2020.00025.

29. Coppola, S., R. Nocerino, L. Paparo, et al. "Therapeutic Effects of Butyrate on Pediatric Obesity: A Randomized Clinical Trial." *JAMA Network Open* 5, no. 12 (December 1, 2022): e2244912. https://doi.org/10.1001/jamanetworkopen.2022.44912.

30. Yano, J. M., K. Yu, G. P. Donaldson, et al. "Indigenous Bacteria from the Gut Microbiota Regulate Host Serotonin Biosynthesis." *Cell* 161, no. 2 (April 9, 2015): 264–76. https://doi.org/10.1016/j.cell.2015.02.047. Erratum in: *Cell* 163 (September 24, 2015): 258. https://doi.org/10.1016/j.cell.2015.09.021.

31. Wikoff, W. R., A. T. Anfora, J. Liu, et al. "Metabolomics Analysis Reveals Large Effects of Gut Microflora on Mammalian Blood Metabolites." *Proceedings of the National Academy of Sciences* 106, no. 10 (March 10, 2009): 3698–703. https://doi.org/10.1073/pnas.0812874106.

32. Cryan, John F., and Timothy G. Dinan. "Talking about a Microbiome Revolution." *Nature Microbiology* 4 (2019): 552–553. https://doi.org/10.1038/s41564-019-0422-9.

33. Hooks, K. B., J. P. Konsman, and M. A. O'Malley. "See the Supplementary Material in Microbiota-Gut-Brain Research: A Critical Analysis." *Behavioral and Brain Sciences* 42 (2019): e60. https://doi.org/10.1017/S0140525X18002133.

34. Johnson, Kevin V., and Kevin R. Foster. "Why Does the Microbiome Affect Behaviour?" *Nature Reviews Microbiology* 16, no. 10 (October 2018): 647–655. https://doi.org/10.1038/s41579-018-0014-3.

35. Parke, Emily C. "Trivial, Interesting, or Overselling? The Microbiome and 'What It Means to Be Human.'" *BioScience* 71, no. 6 (June 2021): 658–663. https://doi.org/10.1093/biosci/biab009.

Chapter 7

1. Ground, W. E. "Causes and Prevention of Puerperal Fever." *The Medical and Surgical Reporter* 73, no. 18 (November 2, 1895).

2. Donovan, William, and Allen McCulloch. "Aseptic Midwifery." *The British Medical Journal* 2, no. 1972 (1898): 1197–98.

3. Döderlein Untersuchungen über das Vorkommen von Spaltpilzen in den Lochien des Uterus und der Vagina gesunder und kranker Wöchnerinnen Archiv für Gynaecologie Bd XXXII S 436. Transted as Döderlein, A. "Investigation of the Occurrence of Fission Fungi in the Lochia of the Uterus and Vagina of Healthy and Sick Women Who Have Recently Given Birth." *Archiv für Gynäkologie* 31 (1887): 412–447. https://doi.org/10.1007/BF01970837.

4. Colebrook, Leonard. "The Prevention of Puerperal Sepsis." *The Journal of Obstetrics and Gynaecology of the British Empire* 43, no. 4 (1936).

5. Colebrook, Leonard. "Prevention of Puerperal Sepsis: A Call to Action." *British Medical Journal* 1, no. 3937 (June 20, 1936): 1257–58. https://doi.org/10.1136/bmj.1.3937.1257.

6. Bohren, M. A., H. Mehrtash, B. Fawole, et al. "How Women Are Treated during Facility-Based Childbirth in Four Countries: A Cross-Sectional Study with Labour Observations and Community-Based Surveys." *The Lancet* 394, no. 10210 (November 9, 2019): 1750–63. https://doi.org/10.1016/S0140-6736(19)31992-0.

7. Zafra-Tanaka, J. H., R. Montesinos-Segura, P. D. Flores-Gonzales, et al. "Potential Excess of Vaginal Examinations during the Management of Labor: Frequency and Associated Factors in 13 Peruvian Hospitals." *Reproductive Health* 16 (2019): 146. https://doi.org/10.1186/s12978-019-0811-9.

8. Cruickshank, R. "Döderlein's Vaginal Bacillus: A Contribution to the Study of the Lacto-Bacilli." *Journal of Hygiene* 31, no. 3 (July 1931): 375–81. https://doi.org/10.1017/S0022172400010901.

9. Johnson, J. L., C. F. Phelps, C. S. Cummins, J. London, and F. Gasser. "Taxonomy of the *Lactobacillus acidophilus* Group." *International Journal of Systematic and Evolutionary Microbiology* 30, no. 1 (1980): 53–68. https://doi.org/10.1099/00207713-30-1-53.

10. Falsen, E., C. Pascual, B. Sjödén, M. Ohlén, and M. D. Collins. "Phenotypic and Phylogenetic Characterization of a Novel *Lactobacillus* Species from Human Sources: Description of *Lactobacillus iners* sp. nov." *International Journal of Systematic Bacteriology* 49, pt. 1 (January 1999): 217–21. https://doi.org/10.1099/00207713-49-1-217.

11. Sobel, J. D. "Is There a Protective Role for Vaginal Flora?" *Current Infectious Disease Reports* 1, no. 4 (October 1999): 379–83. https://doi.org/10.1007/s11908-999-0045-z.

12. Ravel, J., P. Gajer, Z. Abdo, et al. "Vaginal Microbiome of Reproductive-Age Women." *Proceedings of the National Academy of Sciences* 108, Suppl. 1 (March 15, 2011): 4680–87. https://doi.org/10.1073/pnas.1002611107.

13. Barcaite, Egle, Arnoldas Bartusevicius, Rasa Tameliene, et al. "Prevalence of Maternal Group B Streptococcal Colonisation in European Countries." *Acta Obstetricia et Gynecologica Scandinavica* (December 31, 2010). https://doi.org/10.1080/00016340801908759.

14. Gajer, P., R. M. Brotman, G. Bai, et al. "Temporal Dynamics of the Human Vaginal Microbiota." *Science Translational Medicine* 4, no. 132 (May 2, 2012): 132ra52. https://doi.org/10.1126/scitranslmed.3003605.

15. Lebeer, S., S. Ahannach, T. Gehrmann, et al. "A Citizen-Science-Enabled Catalogue of the Vaginal Microbiome and Associated Factors." *Nature Microbiology* 8 (2023): 2183–95. https://doi.org/10.1038/s41564-023-01500-0.

16. Koumans, E. H., M. Sternberg, C. Bruce, et al. "The Prevalence of Bacterial Vaginosis in the United States, 2001–2004; Associations with Symptoms, Sexual Behaviors, and Reproductive Health." *Sexually Transmitted Diseases* 34, no. 11 (November 2007): 864–69. https://doi.org/10.1097/OLQ.0b013e318074e565.

17. Borgdorff, H., C. van der Veer, R. van Houdt, et al. "The Association between Ethnicity and Vaginal Microbiota Composition in Amsterdam, the Netherlands." *PLoS ONE* 12, no. 7 (July 11, 2017): e0181135. https://doi.org/10.1371/journal.pone.0181135.

226 NOTES

18. Srinivasan, S., N. G. Hoffman, M. T. Morgan, et al. "Bacterial Communities in Women with Bacterial Vaginosis: High Resolution Phylogenetic Analyses Reveal Relationships of Microbiota to Clinical Criteria." *PLoS ONE* 7, no. 6 (June 18, 2012): e37818. https://doi.org/10.1371/journal.pone.0037818.
19. Bretelle, F., S. Loubière, R. Desbriere, et al. "Effectiveness and Costs of Molecular Screening and Treatment for Bacterial Vaginosis to Prevent Preterm Birth: The AuTop Randomized Clinical Trial." *JAMA Pediatrics* 177, no. 9 (2023): 894–902. https://doi.org/10.1001/jamapediatrics.2023.2250.

Chapter 8

1. O'Connor, L. E., J. J. Gahche, K. A. Herrick, C. D. Davis, N. Potischman, and A. J. Vargas. "Nonfood Prebiotic, Probiotic, and Synbiotic Use Has Increased in US Adults and Children From 1999 to 2018." *Gastroenterology* 161, no. 2 (August 2021): 476–486.e3. https://doi.org/10.1053/j.gastro.2021.04.037.
2. Gibson, G., R. Hutkins, M. Sanders, et al. "Expert Consensus Document: The International Scientific Association for Probiotics and Prebiotics (ISAPP) Consensus Statement on the Definition and Scope of Prebiotics." *Nature Reviews Gastroenterology & Hepatology* 14 (2017): 491–502. https://doi.org/10.1038/nrgastro.2017.75.
3. Swanson, K. S., G. R. Gibson, R. Hutkins, et al. "The International Scientific Association for Probiotics and Prebiotics (ISAPP) Consensus Statement on the Definition and Scope of Synbiotics." *Nature Reviews Gastroenterology & Hepatology* 17 (2020): 687–701. https://doi.org/10.1038/s41575-020-0344-2.
4. Bindels, L., N. Delzenne, P. Cani, et al. "Towards a More Comprehensive Concept for Prebiotics." *Nature Reviews Gastroenterology & Hepatology* 12 (2015): 303–310. https://doi.org/10.1038/nrgastro.2015.47.
5. Salminen, S., M. C. Collado, A. Endo, et al. "The International Scientific Association of Probiotics and Prebiotics (ISAPP) Consensus Statement on the Definition and Scope of Postbiotics." *Nature Reviews Gastroenterology & Hepatology* 18 (2021): 649–667. https://doi.org/10.1038/s41575-021-00440-6.
6. Donaldson, A.N. "Relation of Constipation to Intestinal Intoxication." *JAMA* 78, no. 12 (1922): 884–888. https://doi.org/10.1001/jama.1922.02640650028011.
7. Metchnikoff, Elie. *The Prolongation of Life: Optimistic Studies.* Translated and edited by P. Chalmers Mitchell. New York and London: The Knickerbocker Press, 1908.
8. The SuDDICU Investigators for the Australian and New Zealand Intensive Care Society Clinical Trials Group. "Effect of Selective Decontamination of the Digestive Tract on Hospital Mortality in Critically Ill Patients Receiving Mechanical Ventilation: A Randomized Clinical Trial." *JAMA* 328, no. 19 (2022): 1911–1921. https://doi.org/10.1001/jama.2022.17927.
9. Centro Sperimental del Latte.
10. McFarland, Lynne V. "From Yaks to Yogurt: The History, Development, and Current Use of Probiotics." *Clinical Infectious Diseases* 60, suppl. 2 (May 2015): S85–S90. https://doi.org/10.1093/cid/civ054.
11. U.S. Department of Health and Human Services, Food and Drug Administration, Centre for Food Safety and Applied Nutrition. "Policy Regarding Quantitative

Labelling of Dietary Supplements Containing Live Microbials: Guidance for Industry." September 2018.

12. Britton, R. A., D. E. Hoffmann, and A. Khoruts. "Probiotics and the Microbiome—How Can We Help Patients Make Sense of Probiotics?" *Gastroenterology* 160, no. 2 (January 2021): 614–623. https://doi.org/10.1053/j.gastro.2020.11.047.

13. Meléndez-Illanes, L., C. González-Díaz, E. Chilet-Rosell, and C. Álvarez-Dardet. "Does the Scientific Evidence Support the Advertising Claims Made for Products Containing *Lactobacillus casei* and *Bifidobacterium lactis*? A Systematic Review." *Journal of Public Health (Oxford)* 38, no. 3 (September 2016): e375–e383. https://doi.org/10.1093/pubmed/fdv151.

14. Lynch, E., J. Troob, B. Lebwohl, and D. E. Freedberg. "Who Uses Probiotics and Why? A Survey Study Conducted among General Gastroenterology Patients." *BMJ Open Gastroenterology* 8, no. 1 (August 2021): e000742. https://doi.org/10.1136/bmjgast-2021-000742.

15. Suez, J., N. Zmora, E. Segal, and E. Elinav. "The Pros, Cons, and Many Unknowns of Probiotics." *Nature Medicine* 25, no. 5 (May 2019): 716–729. https://doi.org/10.1038/s41591-019-0439-x.

16. Su, G. L., C. W. Ko, P. Bercik, et al. "AGA Clinical Practice Guidelines on the Role of Probiotics in the Management of Gastrointestinal Disorders." *Gastroenterology* 159, no. 2 (August 2020): 697–705. https://doi.org/10.1053/j.gastro.2020.05.059.

17. Dethlefsen, L., and D. A. Relman. "Incomplete Recovery and Individualized Responses of the Human Distal Gut Microbiota to Repeated Antibiotic Perturbation." *Proceedings of the National Academy of Sciences* 108, Suppl. 1 (March 15, 2011): 4554–61. https://doi.org/10.1073/pnas.1000087107.

18. Turck, D., J. P. Bernet, J. Marx, et al. "Incidence and Risk Factors of Oral Antibiotic-Associated Diarrhea in an Outpatient Pediatric Population." *Journal of Pediatric Gastroenterology and Nutrition* 37, no. 1 (July 2003): 22–26. https://doi.org/10.1097/00005176-200307000-00004.

19. Guo, Q., J. Z. Goldenberg, C. Humphrey, R. El Dib, and B. C. Johnston. "Probiotics for the Prevention of Pediatric Antibiotic-Associated Diarrhea." *Cochrane Database of Systematic Reviews* 4, no. 4 (April 30, 2019): CD004827. https://doi.org/10.1002/14651858.CD004827.pub5.

20. Vasant, D. H., P. A. Paine, C. J. Black, et al. "British Society of Gastroenterology Guidelines on the Management of Irritable Bowel Syndrome." *Gut* 70, no. 7 (July 2021): 1214–1240. https://doi.org/10.1136/gutjnl-2021-324598.

21. https://www.canada.ca/en/public-health/services/laboratory-biosafety-biosecurity/pathogen-safety-data-sheets-risk-assessment/lactobacillus.html.

22. Zucko, Jurica, Antonio Starcevic, Janko Diminic, et al. "Probiotic—Friend or Foe?" *Current Opinion in Food Science* 32 (2020): 45–49.

23. Bafeta, A., M. Koh, C. Riveros, and P. Ravaud. "Harms Reporting in Randomized Controlled Trials of Interventions Aimed at Modifying Microbiota: A Systematic Review." *Annals of Internal Medicine* 169, no. 4 (August 21, 2018): 240–247. https://doi.org/10.7326/M18-0343.

228 NOTES

24. Yi, S. H., J. A. Jernigan, and L. C. McDonald. "Prevalence of Probiotic Use among Inpatients: A Descriptive Study of 145 U.S. Hospitals." *American Journal of Infection Control* 44, no. 5 (May 1, 2016): 548–553. https://doi.org/10.1016/j.ajic.2015.12.001.

25. Besselink, M. G., H. C. van Santvoort, E. Buskens, et al. "Probiotic Prophylaxis in Predicted Severe Acute Pancreatitis: A Randomised, Double-Blind, Placebo-Controlled Trial." *The Lancet* 371, no. 9613 (February 23, 2008): 651–659. https://doi.org/10.1016/S0140-6736(08)60207-X. Erratum in: *The Lancet* 371, no. 9620 (April 12, 2008): 1246.

26. Yelin, I., K. B. Flett, C. Merakou, et al. "Genomic and Epidemiological Evidence of Bacterial Transmission from Probiotic Capsule to Blood in ICU Patients." *Nature Medicine* 25, no. 11 (November 2019): 1728–1732. https://doi.org/10.1038/s41591-019-0626-9.

27. Kulkarni, T., S. Majarikar, M. Deshmukh, et al. "Probiotic Sepsis in Preterm Neonates—A Systematic Review." *European Journal of Pediatrics* 181 (2022): 2249–2262. https://doi.org/10.1007/s00431-022-04452-5.

28. Oliphant, K., and E. C. Claud. "Early Probiotics Shape Microbiota." *Nature Microbiology* 7, no. 10 (October 2022): 1506–1507. https://doi.org/10.1038/s41564-022-01230-9.

29. https://patient.info/doctor/probiotics-and-prebiotics.

30. Zmora, N., G. Zilberman-Schapira, J. Suez, et al. "Personalized Gut Mucosal Colonization Resistance to Empiric Probiotics Is Associated with Unique Host and Microbiome Features." *Cell* 174, no. 6 (September 6, 2018): 1388–1405.e21. https://doi.org/10.1016/j.cell.2018.08.041.

31. Suez, J., N. Zmora, and E. Elinav. "Probiotics in the Next-Generation Sequencing Era." *Gut Microbes* 11, no. 1 (2020): 77–93. https://doi.org/10.1080/19490976.2019.1586039.

32. Lukasik, J., T. Dierikx, I. Besseling-van der Vaart, et al. "Multispecies Probiotic for the Prevention of Antibiotic-Associated Diarrhea in Children: A Randomized Clinical Trial." *JAMA Pediatrics* 176, no. 9 (September 1, 2022): 860–866. https://doi.org/10.1001/jamapediatrics.2022.1973. Erratum in: *JAMA Pediatrics*, July 5, 2022. https://doi.org/10.1001/jamapediatrics.2022.2351.

33. Allen, S. J., K. Wareham, D. Wang, et al. "Lactobacilli and Bifidobacteria in the Prevention of Antibiotic-Associated Diarrhoea and *Clostridium difficile* Diarrhoea in Older Inpatients (PLACIDE): A Randomised, Double-Blind, Placebo-Controlled, Multicentre Trial." *The Lancet* 382, no. 9900 (October 12, 2013): 1249–1257. https://doi.org/10.1016/S0140-6736(13)61218-0.

34. Suez, J., N. Zmora, G. Zilberman-Schapira, et al. "Post-Antibiotic Gut Mucosal Microbiome Reconstitution Is Impaired by Probiotics and Improved by Autologous FMT." *Cell* 174, no. 6 (September 6, 2018): 1406–1423.e16. https://doi.org/10.1016/j.cell.2018.08.047.

35. Hall, I. C., and E. O'Toole. "Intestinal Flora in New-Born Infants: With a Description of a New Pathogenic Anaerobe, *Bacillus Difficilis*." *American Journal of Diseases of Children* 49, no. 2 (1935): 390–402. https://doi.org/10.1001/archpedi.1935.01970020105010.

Notes 229

36. Eiseman, B., W. Silen, G. S. Bascom, and A. J. Kauvar. "Fecal Enema as an Adjunct in the Treatment of Pseudomembranous Enterocolitis." *Surgery* 44, no. 5 (November 1958): 854–859.
37. National Institute for Health and Care Excellence. "Faecal Microbiota Transplant for Recurrent *Clostridioides difficile* Infection." *Medical Technologies Guidance*, August 31, 2022. https://www.nice.org.uk/guidance/mtg71.
38. Mullish, Benjamin H., M. Nasr Quraishi, James P. Segal, Victoria L. McCune, Matthew Baxter, Gemma L. Marsden, Daniel J. Moore, et al. 2018. "The Use of Faecal Microbiota Transplant as Treatment for Recurrent or Refractory Clostridium difficile Infection and Other Potential Indications: Joint British Society of Gastroenterology (BSG) and Healthcare Infection Society (HIS) Guidelines." Gut 67 (11): 1920–41. https://doi.org/10.1136/gutjnl-2018-316818.
39. Kelly, C. R., E. F. Yen, A. M. Grinspan, et al. "Fecal Microbiota Transplantation Is Highly Effective in Real-World Practice: Initial Results from the FMT National Registry." *Gastroenterology* 160, no. 1 (January 2021): 183–192.e3. https://doi.org/10.1053/j.gastro.2020.09.038.
40. Ekekezie, C., B. K. Perler, A. Wexler, et al. "Understanding the Scope of Do-It-Yourself Fecal Microbiota Transplant." *American Journal of Gastroenterology* 115, no. 4 (April 2020): 603–607. https://doi.org/10.14309/ajg.0000000000000499.
41. Routy, B., J. G. Lenehan, W. H. Miller Jr., et al. "Fecal Microbiota Transplantation Plus Anti-PD-1 Immunotherapy in Advanced Melanoma: A Phase I Trial." *Nature Medicine* 29, no. 8 (August 2023): 2121–2132. https://doi.org/10.1038/s41591-023-02453-x. Erratum in: *Nature Medicine* 30, no. 2 (February 2024): 604. https://doi.org/10.1038/s41591-023-02650-8.
42. Lev-Sagie, A., D. Goldman-Wohl, Y. Cohen, et al. "Vaginal Microbiome Transplantation in Women with Intractable Bacterial Vaginosis." *Nature Medicine* 25, no. 10 (October 2019): 1500–1504. https://doi.org/10.1038/s41591-019-0600-6.
43. Wrønding, T., K. Vomstein, E. F. Bosma, et al. "Antibiotic-Free Vaginal Microbiota Transplant with Donor Engraftment, Dysbiosis Resolution and Live Birth after Recurrent Pregnancy Loss: A Proof-of-Concept Case Study." *EClinicalMedicine* 61 (June 26, 2023): 102070. https://doi.org/10.1016/j.eclinm.2023.102070.
44. Then, C. K., S. Paillas, A. Moomin, et al. "Dietary Fibre Supplementation Enhances Radiotherapy Tumour Control and Alleviates Intestinal Radiation Toxicity." *Microbiome* 12 (2024): 89. https://doi.org/10.1186/s40168-024-01804-1.
45. Louie, T., Y. Golan, S. Khanna, et al. "VE303, a Defined Bacterial Consortium, for Prevention of Recurrent *Clostridioides difficile* Infection: A Randomized Clinical Trial." *JAMA* 329, no. 16 (April 25, 2023): 1356–1366. https://doi.org/10.1001/jama.2023.4314.
46. Mändar, R., G. Sõerunurk, J. Štšepetova, et al. "Impact of *Lactobacillus crispatus*-Containing Oral and Vaginal Probiotics on Vaginal Health: A Randomised Double-Blind Placebo Controlled Clinical Trial." *Beneficial Microbes* 14, no. 2 (April 18, 2023): 143–152. https://doi.org/10.3920/BM2022.0091.

230 NOTES

47. Cohen, P. A. "The Supplement Paradox: Negligible Benefits, Robust Consumption." *JAMA* 316, no. 14 (October 11, 2016): 1453–1454. https://doi.org/10.1001/jama.2016.14252.

Chapter 9

1. Whittaker, R. H. *Vegetation of the Siukiyou Mountains, Oregon and California.* First published October 1, 1960. https://doi.org/10.2307/1948435.
2. Aagaard, K., J. Petrosino, W. Keitel, M. Watson, J. Katancik, N. Garcia, S. Patel, et al. "The Human Microbiome Project Strategy for Comprehensive Sampling of the Human Microbiome and Why It Matters." *FASEB Journal* 27, no. 3 (March 2013): 1012–22. https://doi.org/10.1096/fj.12-220806.
3. Stephens, A., and A. Kozik. "Psychosocial Stress and the Gut Microbiota." *Nature Microbiology* 7 (2022): 1505. https://doi.org/10.1038/s41564-022-01225-6.
4. Delgado, A. Nieves, and J. Baedke. "Does the Human Microbiome Tell Us Something about Race?" *Humanities and Social Sciences Communications* 8 (2021): 97. https://doi.org/10.1057/s41599-021-00772-3.
5. Allali, I., R. E. Abotsi, L. A. Tow, L. Thabane, H. J. Zar, N. M. Mulder, and M. P. Nicol. "Human Microbiota Research in Africa: A Systematic Review Reveals Gaps and Priorities for Future Research." *Microbiome* 9, no. 1 (December 15, 2021): 241. https://doi.org/10.1186/s40168-021-01195-7. Erratum in: *Microbiome* 10, no. 1 (January 19, 2022): 10. https://doi.org/10.1186/s40168-021-01212-9.
6. Mangola, S. M., J. R. Lund, S. L. Schnorr, et al. "Ethical Microbiome Research with Indigenous Communities." *Nature Microbiology* 7 (2022): 749–756. https://doi.org/10.1038/s41564-022-01116-w.
7. Good, Kenneth, and David Chanoff. *Into the Heart: One Man's Pursuit of Love and Knowledge Among the Yanomami.* Pearson, 1997.
8. De Filippo, C., D. Cavalieri, M. Di Paola, M. Ramazzotti, J. B. Poullet, S. Massart, S. Collini, G. Pieraccini, and P. Lionetti. "Impact of Diet in Shaping Gut Microbiota Revealed by a Comparative Study in Children from Europe and Rural Africa." *Proceedings of the National Academy of Sciences of the United States of America* 107, no. 33 (2010): 14691–96. https://doi.org/10.1073/pnas.1005963107.
9. Crittenden, A. N., and S. L. Schnorr. "Current Views on Hunter-Gatherer Nutrition and the Evolution of the Human Diet." *American Journal of Physical Anthropology* 162 (2017): 84–109. https://doi.org/10.1002/ajpa.23148.
10. Yatsunenko, T., F. Rey, M. Manary, et al. "Human Gut Microbiome Viewed Across Age and Geography." *Nature* 486 (2012): 222–27. https://doi.org/10.1038/nature11053.
11. Merrill, B. D., M. M. Carter, M. R. Olm, D. Dahan, S. Tripathi, S. P. Spencer, B. Yu, et al. "Ultra-Deep Sequencing of Hadza Hunter-Gatherers Recovers Vanishing Gut Microbes." *bioRxiv* (2022). https://doi.org/10.1101/2022.03.30.486478.
12. Fragiadakis, G. K., S. A. Smits, E. D. Sonnenburg, W. Van Treuren, G. Reid, R. Knight, A. Manjurano, et al. "Links Between Environment, Diet, and the Hunter-Gatherer Microbiome." *Gut Microbes* 10, no. 2 (2019): 216–27. https://doi.org/10.1080/19490976.2018.1494103.

Notes 231

13. Girard, C., N. Tromas, M. Amyot, and B. J. Shapiro. "Gut Microbiome of the Canadian Arctic Inuit." *mSphere* 2 (2017). https://doi.org/10.1128/msphere.00297-16.
14. Keohane, D. M., T. S. Ghosh, I. B. Jeffery, et al. "Microbiome and Health Implications for Ethnic Minorities After Enforced Lifestyle Changes." *Nature Medicine* 26 (2020): 1089–95. https://doi.org/10.1038/s41591-020-0963-8.
15. Ayeni, F. A., E. Biagi, S. Rampelli, J. Fiori, M. Soverini, H. J. Audu, S. Cristino, et al. "Infant and Adult Gut Microbiome and Metabolome in Rural Bassa and Urban Settlers from Nigeria." *Cell Reports* 23, no. 10 (2018): 3056–67. https://doi.org/10.1016/j.celrep.2018.05.018.
16. Vangay, P., A. J. Johnson, T. L. Ward, G. A. Al-Ghalith, R. R. Shields-Cutler, B. M. Hillmann, S. K. Lucas, et al. "US Immigration Westernizes the Human Gut Microbiome." *Cell* 175, no. 4 (2018): 962–972.e10. https://doi.org/10.1016/j.cell.2018.10.029.
17. Santiago-Rodriguez, T. M., G. Fornaciari, S. Luciani, S. E. Dowd, G. A. Toranzos, I. Marota, and R. J. Cano. "Gut Microbiome of an 11th Century A.D. Pre-Columbian Andean Mummy." *PLoS ONE* 10, no. 9 (2015): e0138135. https://doi.org/10.1371/journal.pone.0138135.
18. Wibowo, M. C., Z. Yang, M. Borry, et al. "Reconstruction of Ancient Microbial Genomes from the Human Gut." *Nature* 594 (2021): 234–39. https://doi.org/10.1038/s41586-021-03532-0.
19. Rampelli, S., S. Turroni, C. Mallol, et al. "Components of a Neanderthal Gut Microbiome Recovered from Fecal Sediments from El Salt." *Communications Biology* 4 (2021): 169. https://doi.org/10.1038/s42003-021-01689-y.
20. Moeller, A. H., Y. Li, E. Mpoudi Ngole, S. Ahuka-Mundeke, E. V. Lonsdorf, A. E. Pusey, M. Peeters, B. H. Hahn, and H. Ochman. "Rapid Changes in the Gut Microbiome During Human Evolution." *Proceedings of the National Academy of Sciences of the United States of America* 111, no. 46 (2014): 16431–35. https://doi.org/10.1073/pnas.1419136111.
21. Ley, R. E., M. Hamady, C. Lozupone, P. J. Turnbaugh, R. R. Ramey, J. S. Bircher, M. L. Schlegel, et al. "Evolution of Mammals and Their Gut Microbes." *Science* 320, no. 5883 (2008): 1647–51. https://doi.org/10.1126/science.1155725. Erratum in: *Science* 322, no. 5905 (November 21, 2008): 1188. https://doi.org/10.1126/science.322.5905.1188-a.
22. Nishida, A. H., and H. Ochman. "Rates of Gut Microbiome Divergence in Mammals." *Molecular Ecology* 27, no. 8 (2018): 1884–97. https://doi.org/10.1111/mec.14473.
23. Burkitt, D. P. "Epidemiology of Large Bowel Disease: The Role of Fibre." *Proceedings of the Nutrition Society* 32, no. 3 (1973): 145–49. https://doi.org/10.1079/pns19730032.
24. Blackley, Charles Harrison. *Experimental Researches on the Causes and Nature of Catarrhus Aestivus.* London: Balliere, Tindall and Cox, 1873.
25. Floyer, John. *A Treatise of the Asthma. Divided into Four Parts.* 2nd ed. London: R. Wilkin, 1717.

232 NOTES

26. Russell, G. "The Childhood Asthma Epidemic." *Thorax* 61, no. 4 (2006): 276–78. https://doi.org/10.1136/thx.2005.052662.
27. Barker, D. J. P., C. Osmond, J. Golding, and M. E. J. Wadsworth. "Acute Appendicitis and Bathrooms in Three Samples of British Children." *BMJ* 296 (April 2, 1988).
28. Strachan, D. P. "Hay Fever, Hygiene, and Household Size." *BMJ* 299, no. 6710 (1989): 1259–60. https://doi.org/10.1136/bmj.299.6710.1259.
29. von Mutius, E., and S. Schmid. "The PASTURE Project: EU Support for the Improvement of Knowledge About Risk Factors and Preventive Factors for Atopy in Europe." *Allergy* 61 (2006): 407–13. https://doi.org/10.1111/j.1398-9995.2006. 01009.x.
30. von Mutius, E. "The 'Hygiene Hypothesis' and PASTURE Project: EU Support Studies." *Frontiers in Immunology* 12 (2021): 63522. https://doi.org/10.3389/fimmu. 2021.635522.
31. Blaser, M. J. "The Theory of Disappearing Microbiota and the Epidemics of Chronic Diseases." *Nature Reviews Immunology* 17, no. 8 (2017): 461–63. https://doi. org/10.1038/nri.2017.77.
32. Sonnenburg, E. D., and J. L. Sonnenburg. "The Ancestral and Industrialized Gut Microbiota and Implications for Human Health." *Nature Reviews Microbiology* 17 (2019): 383–90. https://doi.org/10.1038/s41579-019-0191-8.
33. Tomova, A., I. Bukovsky, E. Rembert, W. Yonas, J. Alwarith, N. D. Barnard, and H. Kahleova. "The Effects of Vegetarian and Vegan Diets on Gut Microbiota." *Frontiers in Nutrition* 6 (2019): 47. https://doi.org/10.3389/fnut.2019.00047.
34. Barone, M., S. Turroni, S. Rampelli, M. Soverini, F. D'Amico, E. Biagi, P. Brigidi, E. Troiani, and M. Candela. "Gut Microbiome Response to a Modern Paleolithic Diet in a Western Lifestyle Context." *PLoS ONE* 14, no. 8 (2019): e0220619. https:// doi.org/10.1371/journal.pone.0220619.
35. David, L. A., C. F. Maurice, R. N. Carmody, et al. "Diet Rapidly and Reproducibly Alters the Human Gut Microbiome." *Nature* 505 (2014): 559–63. https://doi.org/10. 1038/nature12820.
36. Kuehnast, T., C. Abbott, M. R. Pausan, et al. "The Crewed Journey to Mars and Its Implications for the Human Microbiome." *Microbiome* 10 (2022): 26. https://doi.org/ 10.1186/s40168-021-01222-7.

Conclusion

1. Natalini, J. G., S. Singh, and L. N. Segal. "The Dynamic Lung Microbiome in Health and Disease." *Nature Reviews Microbiology* 21, no. 4 (2023): 222–235. https:// doi.org/10.1038/s41579-022-00821-x.
2. Berg, G., D. Rybakova, D. Fischer, T. Cernava, M. C. Vergès, T. Charles, X. Chen, et al. "Microbiome Definition Re-Visited: Old Concepts and New Challenges." *Microbiome* 8, no. 1 (2020): 103. https://doi.org/10.1186/s40168-020-00875-0. *Erratum in*: Microbiome. 2020 Aug 20;8(1):119. https://doi.org/10.1186/s40168-020-00905-x.

3. Hammer, Tobin J., Jon G. Sanders, and Noah Fierer. "Not All Animals Need a Microbiome." *FEMS Microbiology Letters* 366, no. 10 (May 2019): fnz117. https://doi.org/10.1093/femsle/fnz117.
4. Walker, A. W., and L. Hoyles. "Human Microbiome Myths and Misconceptions." *Nature Microbiology* 8 (2023): 1392–1396. https://doi.org/10.1038/s41564-023-01426-7.
5. Boers, S. A., R. Jansen, and J. P. Hays. "Suddenly Everyone Is a Microbiota Specialist." *Clinical Microbiology and Infection* 22, no. 7 (July 2016): 581–582. https://doi.org/10.1016/j.cmi.2016.05.002.
6. Douglas, A. E., and J. H. Werren. "Holes in the Hologenome: Why Host-Microbe Symbioses Are Not Holobionts." *mBio* 7, no. 2 (March 31, 2016): e02099-15. https://doi.org/10.1128/mBio.02099-15.
7. Johnson, K. V. A., and K. R. Foster. "Why Does the Microbiome Affect Behaviour?" *Nature Reviews Microbiology* 16 (2018): 647–655. https://doi.org/10.1038/s41579-018-0014-3.
8. Parke, Emily C. "Trivial, Interesting, or Overselling? The Microbiome and 'What It Means to Be Human.'" *BioScience* 71, no. 6 (June 2021): 658–663. https://doi.org/10.1093/biosci/biab009.
9. O'Toole, P. W., and M. Paoli. "The Human Microbiome, Global Health and the Sustainable Development Goals: Opportunities and Challenges." *Nature Reviews Microbiology* 21, no. 10 (October 2023): 624–625. https://doi.org/10.1038/s41579-023-00924-z.

INDEX

For the benefit of digital users, indexed terms that span two pages (e.g., 52–53) may, on occasion, appear on only one of those pages.

Page numbers followed by *f* indicate figures.

16S rRNA sequencing, 32–35, 37, 97–98
18S rRNA, 33

A

AAD (antibiotic-associated diarrhea), 172–174, 177, 178
ABI 3730XL DNA sequencing, 34
Acinetobacter, 83, 101, 103
Adenovirus, 10*f*
adipose tissue, 42
adrenal glands, 116, 120, 128–131
Aeromonas, 101
affluence, diseases of, 195, 198–199
AGA (American Gastroenterological Association), 172
agar gel, 46
Agta people, 189
air purity, 22–23
air quality, 22–23
Akkermansia muciniphila, 113
Alcaligenes, 101
alcohol gel hand sanitizers, 59–60
ALEX group (the Allergy and Endotoxin study), 200
algae, 5–6, 7*f*, 21, 23

Alistipes onderdonkii, 105–106
Alistipes putredinis, 105–106
Alistipes shahii, 105–106
allergies, 73–74, 196, 199–200
alpha diversity, 184
Amazonas State, Venezuela, 189
American diet, 100
American Gastroenterological Association (AGA), 172
American Gut Project, 105
Amici, Giovanni Battista, 9–11
Amsel's criteria, 158–159
anaerobes
  facultative, 65
  in milk-fed stools, 69
  transfer from mother to baby, 74–75
  in vaginal microbiome, 153
ancient Greece, 197–198
ancient microbiota, 192
animalcules, 9–10, 12
animals, 5, 108–109
  germ-free, 26–28, 109–111, 134
  survival without a microbiome, 26–27
anthrax, 14
anthrax bacillus, 14
antibacterial soap products, 60

antibiotic-associated diarrhea
(AAD), 172–174, 177, 178
antibiotics, 18–19, 58, 60, 131–132, 149,
160, 201–202
antidepressants, 134
antiseptics, 18–19, 60, 141
ants, omnivorous, 108–109
anxiety, 115–116, 118
appendicitis, 196, 199–200
archaea, 32–33
in gut microbiome, 93–94
in skin microbiome, 48
archaeological samples, 192
Aristotle, 20–21
aseptic technique(s), 139–142, 149
Aspergillus, 48
asthma, 73, 196, 197–199
atopic dermatitis, 63
atopy, 198–199
Austria, 200
autoinfection, 141–142, 146–148
autointoxication, 164–165

B
BaAka rainforest hunter-gatherers, 189
babies
breech, 78
newborn, 64, 66*f*
premature, 175–176
bacilli (term), 11
Bacillus bifidus communis, 70
Bacillus difficile, 179
Bacillus pyocyaneus, 56
Bacillus subtilis, 70
back-breeding, 123–124
bacteria, 4, 6–7, 9, 9*f*, 23, 32
anaerobic, 65, 69, 74–75, 153
archaebacteria, 32
avirulent, 13
in babies, 70–72
bifidobacteria, 83–85, 145–146

comma-shaped, 12
commensal, 13
extremophiles, 32
fecal, 143
food, 100, 103
Gram-negative, 46–47
Gram-positive, 46–48, 145*f*
in gut, 86–87, 90–94, 99–100, 107, 111
intestinal (enteric), 93
maternal gut-utero axis, 77
in milk-fed babies, 69
number consumed daily, 100
number inside us, 2
in ocean, 23–24
in penis, 156
placenta, 75–76
rod-shaped, 11
size of, 8
in skin, 45–52
in soil, 25
spread from toilets, 102–103
in stool, 72, 83, 91, 103, 111–112
terminology, 12
transfer from mother to baby, 74–75
vaginal, 71–72, 142–143
vegetative, 13
bacterial colonies, 46
Bacterial and Viral Bioinformatics Resource
Centre (BV-BRC), 49
bacterial vaginosis (BV), 158–160
Amsel's criteria for, 158–159
Nugent's criteria for, 158–159
treatment of, 181–182
bacteriophages, 7
in gut, 94
in ocean, 24
in skin, 48
Bacterium coli commune, 69
Bacteroides, 86–87, 91, 103, 106, 156–157,
187–188, 190, 191, 193
Bacteroides thetaiotaomicron, 113

236 INDEX

Bacteroides uniformis, 105–106
Bacteroides vulgatus, 105–106
Bacteroidetes, 93, 192
Baird, Spencer F., 12
BALB/c mice, 124–125, 127–129
Bangladesh, 186
Beauveria bassiana, 14
benign commensals, 49
Bermuda Institute of Ocean Science
  (BIOS), 34–35
beta diversity, 184
beta-naphthol, 165
bifidobacteria, 83–85, 106–107, 145–146,
  169, 187
Bifidobacterium, 86–87, 91–93, 103,
  127–128, 171, 192
Bifidobacterium adolescentis, 70–71
Bifidobacterium bifidum, 70–71
Bifidobacterium breve, 70–71
Bifidobacterium longum, 70–71
Bill and Melinda Gates Foundation, 186
bioaerosol, 21–24
biomes, 2–3
BIOS (Bermuda Institute of Ocean
  Science), 34–35
Black Death, 15
Blackley, Charles Harrison, 196–197
Blastocystis, 94
Botrytis bassiana, 14
bottled water, 102
Boulard, Henri, 169
Boulpon, Burkina Faso, 187–188
brain, 115
  gut-brain axis, 117–118–119*f*, 122–123,
    130–133
  gut microbiome and, 115–117
  microbiome-gut-brain studies in
    mice, 127–130
breastfeeding, 85
breast milk, 84
breech babies, 78

British Agricultural Revolution, 24–25
Bulgarian bacillus, 166–167
Burkina Faso, 187–188
butyrate, 132
BV. *see* bacterial vaginosis
BV-BRC (Bacterial and Viral Bioinformatics
  Resource Centre), 49

C

caesarean-born babies
  bacteria of, 72–73
  health differences in, 73–74
Callidusccus callidus, 192
calorie intake, 107–108
calprotectin, fecal, 82–83
Cambodia, 186
Canada: microbiome projects in, 39
Canadian Arctic people, 190
Candida, 48, 94, 100
Candida albicans, 57–58, 86–87
carnivores, 109, 194
centenarians, 166
CFU (colony forming unit), 55
Chadwick, Edwin, 15–16
checkpoint inhibitor chemotherapy, 181
Chemin, M., 166
chemotherapy, 181
Chepang people, 189
childbirth, 139–142
children
  antibiotic-associated diarrhea (AAD)
    in, 173
  asthma in, 73
  caesarean-born, 73
  on farms, 200
  malnourished, 111–112
  in urban *vs* rural areas, 187–188
Chlorella, 7*f*
chlorophyll, 6, 7*f*
chloroplasts, 5
cholera, 15, 101–102

Index 237

citizen science, 154–155
Cladosporium, 94
cleanliness, 4–5, 58, 139–141
Clostridium, 86–87, 91–93, 103, 192
Clostridium difficile, 59, 212
  commensal, 182
Clostridium difficile infection, 178–180
cocci (term), 11
Cochrane group, 172–174
Colebrook, Dora, 147–148
Colebrook, Leonard, 147–149
colic, 82–83
Colobus monkeys, 194
colon (large intestine), 91, 92*f*, 107
colonization resistance, 50, 69, 145–146
colony forming unit (CFU), 55
Comamonas, 101
commercial stool tests, 87
common core, 106
communities (term), 210
community state types (CST), 153–154
contagion theory, 14–16
contraception, 4
coprolites (fossilized stool), 192
core mammalian microbiome, 194
core microbiome, 105–107
corneocytes, 42–43, 45
cortisol, 120–121
Corynebacterium, 47–48, 53–54, 73, 86–87, 156–157
costs, 186, 209
counting microbes, 209
Crimean War (1854), 16
Crohn's disease, 172, 198–199
cryptogamia, 13, 18
cryptogamic flora, 61–62
culturomics, 96–98, 208–209
Cutibacterium (formerly known as *Propionibacterium*), 47–48
Cutibacterium acnes, 156–157

D

DACC (Data Analysis and Coordination Centre), 38–39
Darwin, Charles, 21
Data Analysis and Coordination Centre (DACC), 38–39
DBA/2J mice, 123–124
Debaryomyces, 100
decontamination, 57–58, 167
  selective, 165
deep sequencing, 36
depression, 133–135
dermatitis, atopic, 63
dermatological problems, 61–63
dermis, 42, 44
diarrhoea, 15
  antibiotic-associated (AAD), 172–174, 177, 178
dietary measures
  American diet, 100
  loss of microbiome diversity and, 204–205
  low microbiota-accessible-carbohydrate (MAC) diet, 111
  Paleolithic diets, 205
  probiotics and, 167
  US Department of Agriculture–recommended diet, 100
  Western diet, 187
dietary nutrients, 103
digestion, 121–122
disease(s)
  of affluence, 195, 198–199
  contagion theory of, 14–16
  germ theory of, 14–19
  infectious, 15–17, 202–203
  loss of microbiome diversity and, 195–198
diversity, 211
  alpha, 184, 191

238 INDEX

diversity (*Continued*)
  beta, 184
  definition of, 184–185, 210
  differences in, 190–191
  ethnocultural, 185
  and health, 195–198
  in hunter-gatherers, 188–190
  past, 192
  of research, 185–186
  rewilding, 203–206
  in rural areas, 187–188
  in stool microbiomes, 186
  in urban areas, 187–188
DNA sequencing, 34
  16S rRNA, 32–35, 37
  ABI 3730XL, 34
  high-throughput, 36
  massively parallel, 36
  metagenomic, 34–37
  nanopore, 37
  next-generation, 36
  Pyrosequencing 454, 35
  second-generation, 36
Doderlein, Albert, 142–147, 150–151
Doderlein's bacillus, 144–145
drinking water, 101–102
Ducleux, Emile, 17
dust particles, 21–22, 200
Dutch Microbiome Project, 104
dynamic microbiomes, 208
dysbiosis, 159

E
East Africa, 196
eczema, 62–63, 196, 199
Eden Project, 2
Eggerthella, 153
Ehrenberg, Christian Gottfried, 11–13, 21
Eiseman, B., 179
Elevated Plus Maze test, 125, 129
Elevated Zero Maze test, 125

endocrine system, 120–122
engrafting, 167–168, 177
Enhydrobacter aerosaccus, 47–48
Entamoeba, 94
enteric system, 120–122
Enterobacter, 60, 101
Enterobacteriaceae, 91–93
enterochromaffin cells, 121, 133
Enterococcus, 57–58, 86–87, 103
Enterococcus avium, 156
Enterococcus faecalis, 70, 156
entophytes, 12–13, 18
entozoa, 12
environmental microbiome, 20–21
environmental research, 31–33
epidermis, 42–43*f*, 43
erythema toxicum neonatorum, 66–67
Escherich, Theodore, 67–69, 211
Escherichia coli, 34, 69–70, 93, 127–128, 156–157, 169
esophagus, 90–91
ethnocultural diversity, 185
Eubacterium rectale, 105–106
Eukaryotes, 23, 32
Europe
  allergic disease in children studies, 200
  microbiome projects, 39
Euryarchaeota, 48
evolution, 135–137, 193–194
extremophiles, 32

F
facultative anaerobes, 65
Faecalibacterium, 192
Faecalibacterium prausnitzii, 105–106
family size, 199–200
farm children, 200
fecal bacteria, 143
fecal calprotectin, 82–83
fecal microbiota transplants (FMTs), 178, 180, 181

definition of, 178
do-it-yourself (DIY), 180–181, 186
guidelines for, 180
National Registry for FMTs, 180
female urethra, 157
fermented foods, 162–163, 165–167
fetal meconium, 78–79
fetal microbiome, 81–83
fiber intake, 112–114, 181, 187, 205
Finland, 200
Firmicutes, 93
Flavobacterium, 101
Florence, Italy, 187
flow cytometry, 209
Floyer, John, 197–198
fluoxetine (Prozac), 133
FMTs. *see* fecal microbiota transplants
food(s)
  fermented, 162–163, 165–167
  Ready to Use Supplementary Food
    (RUSF), 112
  refeeding formulations, 112
food absorption, 109–111
Food and Drug Administration (FDA), 58,
  170
food bacteria, 100, 103
food preparation, 4–5
Forced Swimming Test, 125–126
fossilized stool (coprolites), 192
Fox, John, 15
functional core, 108
fungi, 14
  in gut, 86–87, 94, 100
  microscopic, 5, 6*f*
  mycorrhizal, 25
  in ocean, 23
  in skin, 48, 61–62
  vaginal, 142–143
future directions of the mi-
    crobiome, 181–182,
    206–207

G

Gardnerella, 153
Gardnerella vaginalis, 158
gastroenteritis, 68, 173
gastrointestinal tract, 88–91
generally recognized as safe (GRAS)
    status, 170–171, 174
genital tract microbes. *see also* vaginal
    microbiome(s)
  importance of, 138–139
  male genital microbiome, 156–157
gentian-violet, 46–47
Germany, 200
germ-free animals, 130, 134
  food absorption by, 109–111
  gut-brain axis in, 122–123
  housing for, 27–28
  survival of, 26–27, 31
germ-free environments, 26–27
germ-free humans, 29–31
germ-free research, 29, 31
germs, 3–4
germ theory, 14–19, 212
Ghahibo Amerindians, 189
glans penis, 156–157
glossopharyngeal nerve, 119*f*
"The Golden Snuffbox," 20–21
gonorrhea, 143
Good, David, 186
Good, Kenneth, 186
Grammatophora oceanica, 21
Gram-negative organisms, 46–48
Gram-positive bacteria, 46–48, 145*f*
Gram-stain, 46–47
GRAS (generally recognized as safe)
    status, 170–171, 174
great apes, 193
Grigoroff, M., 166
Ground, William E., 146–147
gut-brain axis, 117–118–119*f*, 118–122
  in germ-free mice, 122–123

240 INDEX

gut-brain axis (*Continued*)
  microbiome-gut-brain studies, 127–130
  microbes and, 135–137
  microbial metabolites and, 131–133
  microbiome-gut-brain axis, 118
GutFeelingKB, 105–106
gut microbiome, 86
  brain and, 115–117
  calorie intake and, 107–108
  dietary nutrients and, 103
  fiber intake and, 112–114
  gut-brain axis direction by, 130–131
  loss of microbes from, 111–112
  manipulation of, 164–167
  microbes in, 91–94, 103–105
  of newborn babies, 83
  number of bacteria in, 2
  number of microbes consumed
    daily, 100
  as open ecosystem, 98–100, 194
  reliability of research on, 94–98
  variability of, 103–105
Gut Microbiome Health Index, 105–106
gut tests, 86–87

H

Hadza people, 189–190, 205
hair follicles, 43*f*, 44
Hall, Ivan C., 70
Halomonas, 78–79
hands
  as key transmitters of skin
    microbiome, 52–54
  skin microbiome of, 53–56
hand soaps, 2
hand sterilizer, 57–61
handwashing, 4, 139
  in childbirth, 139, 141
  effects on skin microbiome, 54–57,
    60–61
  with soap *vs* hand sterilizer, 57–61

WHO guidelines for, 58–59
HART (highly active anti-retroviral
  treatment), 153
Harvard Bussey Institute, 123–124
Hawaii Space Exploration Analog and
  Simulation IV, 206–207
Hay bacillus, 70
hay fever, 196–197, 199, 200
health
  changes in microbiome diversity
    and, 195–198
  intestinal, 86
  mental, 30–31, 115
  public, 15–16
healthcare workers, 57–58
herbivores, 109, 193–194
Hexamitidae, 94
highly active anti-retroviral treatment
  (HART), 153
high-throughput DNA sequencing, 36
Himalayas, 191
history
  first description of the
    microbiome, 12–13
  first-ever probiotic, 166–167, 169
  first person to *see* microbes, 9–12
  past diversity, 192
HIV infection, 50, 153
HMOs (human milk
  oligosaccharides), 84–85
HMP (Human Microbiome Project), 38–40
HMP1 (2008 to 2012), 38–39
host-adapted core, 106–107
HPA (hypothalamic-pituitary-adrenal)
  axis, 116, 120, 128–131
Human Genome Project, 37
Human Microbiome Project
  (HMP), 37–40, 103–104, 185
  HMP1 (2008 to 2012), 38–39
  integrated HMP (iHMP, 2013 to
    2016), 38–39

Index 241

human milk oligosaccharides (HMOs), 84–85
human papillomavirus, 48
Human Phenotype Project, 105
hunter-gatherers, 186, 188–191, 193, 195, 202–203
hygiene, 4–5, 16, 18–19
hygiene hypothesis, 73–74, 198–203
hypothalamic-pituitary-adrenal (HPA) axis, 116, 120, 128–131

I

ICNP (International Code of Nomenclature of Prokaryotes), 95
iHMP (integrated HMP, 2013 to 2016), 38–39
Illumina, 35
immigrants from Thailand, 191
immune-modulating chemotherapy, 181
immunology, 201
India, 196
infant mortality, 67–68
infants
  gastroenteritis infections in, 68
  newborn babies, 64, 66*f*
infant stool, 70–72, 84
infectious disease(s), 15–17, 202–203
  autoinfection, 141–142, 146–148
  causes of, 149–150
  Clostridium difficile infection, 178–180
  HIV, 153
  infant gastroenteritis infections, 68
  post-puerperal infection, 147–149
  probiotic sepsis, 175–176
  sexual infections, 156
  skin infections, 50
infertility treatment, 181
infusoria, 12–13, 21
integrated HMP (iHMP, 2013 to 2016), 38–39

International Code of Nomenclature of Prokaryotes (ICNP), 95
International Scientific Association for Probiotics and Prebiotics, 161–162
intestinal flora, 13
intestinal health, 86
intestinal tract, 88–91
Ion Torrent, 35
Irish travelers, 190–191
irritable bowel syndrome, 118, 174
ISALA study, 154–155

J

Jackson Labs, 124
Jantet, Ambroise, 166
Japan
  microbiome projects, 39
  neonatal research, 70–71
Julus marginatus, 12–13

K

keratinization, 42
keratinocytes, 42–43, 45
key microbes, 105–107, 150–152
kitome, 77
Klebsiella, 93, 101, 156–157
Klebsiella pneumoniae, 60
Koch, Robert, 14, 62, 67, 101–102
Koch's postulates, 18

L

lab mice, 123–127
lactobacilli, 145*f*, 145–146, 150–154, 177
Lactobacillus, 53, 86–87, 91–93, 100, 171
Lactobacillus acidophilus, 70, 144–145, 150–151
Lactobacillus amylovorus, 151
Lactobacillus casei Shirota strain, 169
Lactobacillus crispatus, 151, 153, 182
Lactobacillus crispii, 212

242 INDEX

Lactobacillus delbrueckii subspecies *Bulgaricus*, 166–167, 169
Lactobacillus gallinarum, 151
Lactobacillus gasseri, 151, 153
Lactobacillus helveticus, 169
Lactobacillus iners, 151, 153, 154–155
Lactobacillus jensenii, 153
Lactobacillus johnsonii, 151
Lactobacillus reuteri, 169
Lactobacillus rhamnosus, 169–170, 173
Lactobacillus rhamnosus GG, 169, 175
Lactococcus, 171
Lactococcus lactis, 100, 169–170
Lancefield, Rebecca, 147
Lancefield Group A streptococcus, 147–148
Langerhans cells, 42
Langur monkeys, 194
large intestine (colon), 91–92f, 91, 107
Lawrence, Raymond J., 29–30
Leach, Jeff D., 186
Leeuwenhoek, Antonie van, 9–10
Leidy, Joseph, 12–13, 18, 21
Leishmania mexicana, 8f
lifestyle factors, 154–155, 202–203
Lister, Joseph (Sr.), 10–11
Lister, Joseph Jackson, 10–11
Little, Clarence C., 123–124
live biotherapeutic products (LBPs), 182, 212
longevity, 166
low microbiota-accessible-carbohydrate (MAC) diet, 111
low- or no-biomass research, 77–80
lymph nodes, 80–81

M

Malassezia, 48, 61–62
Malawi, 189, 193

MALDI-TOF (Matrix-Assisted Laser Desorption Ionization Time-Of-Flight) mass spectrometry, 97
male genital microbiome, 156–157
male urethra, 157–158
malnutrition, 111–112
mammals, other, 193–194
Marc, Nicole, 166
Mars, 2–3
Mars500 project, 206
maternal gut-utero axis, 77
Matrix-Assisted Laser Desorption Ionization Time-Of-Flight (MALDI-TOF) mass spectrometry, 97
meat, 103
meconium, 68–70
fetal, 78–79
Medawar, Peter, 7–8
melanocytes, 42
mental health, 30–31
mental health disorders, 115
Merkel Cell polyomavirus, 48
metabolic system, 121–122
metabolites, microbial, 131–133
metabolomics, 36
metagenomics, 38, 77–78, 94, 97–98, 185, 208–209
costs of, 186, 209
vs culturomics, 97
low- or no-biomass research, 79–80
on probiotics, 176–178
research techniques, 95–97, 176
metagenomic sequencing, 35–37
shotgun, 34–35
metaproteomics, 36
metatranscriptomics, 36
Metchnikoff, Elie, 164–167, 176, 177
Methanobrevibacter, 193
Methanobrevibacter smithii, 93–94
Methanomicrobiales, 32–33

Index   243

methicillin-resistant *Staphylococcus aureus* (MRSA), 49–51, 57–58
mice
  germ-free, 122–123, 130
  microbiome-gut-brain studies in, 127–130
  lab, 123–127
microbe (term), 12
microbes
  ancient, 192
  classification of, 11–13
  counting, 209
  definition of, 5–9
  and depression, 133–135
  description of, 12
  evolution of, 135–137, 193
  first person to *see* microbes, 9–12
  genital tract, 138–139
  gut, 91–94, 103–105, 164–167
  and gut-brain axis, 135–137
  loss from our gut, 111–112
  number consumed daily, 100
  in penis microbiome, 156–157
  probiotic examples, 168–169
  size of, 8–9
  in stool samples, 91–93
  in tap water, 101–102
  in vaginal microbiome, 144–145, 145*f*, 147–154
microbe supplements, 112
microbial metabolites, 131–133
microbiology, 9–10
microbiome(s), 208
  ancient, 192
  and the brain, 115
  change over time, 68–69
  core mammalian, 194
  definition of, 1–3, 208
  diverse, 211
  dynamic, 208
  environmental, 20–21

  evolution of, 193–194
  fetal, 81–83
  first description of, 12–13
  future, 206–207
  and the genitals, 138
  gut, 86, 117–118
  Human Microbiome Project (HMP), 37–40
  in hunter-gatherers, 188–190
  importance of, 3–5
  locations of, 20
  male genital, 156–157
  of newborn babies, 64
  normal, 103–104
  ocean, 23–24
  penis, 156–157
  placental, 75–76
  removal of, 25–26
  research projects, 39
  rewilding, 203–206
  in rural areas, 187–188
  skin, 41
  soil, 24–25
  survival without, 26–27
  testicular, 158
  translational science, 39–40
  in urban areas, 187–188
  urethral, 158
  vaginal, 142–143, 145*f*, 152–155
  variability of, 45–46, 103–105, 211
microbiome diversity
  differences in, 190–191
  and health, 195–198
  loss of, 184
  past, 192
microbiome-gut-brain axis, 118, 127–130
microbiome industry, 161
Microbiomejournal, 164
MicrobiomePost, 164
microbiome research. *see* research
Micrococcus, 78–79

244 INDEX

microflora, 13
micronutrients, 110
microscopes, 9–11, 97–98
Middle Ages, 20–21, 197–198
milk-fed babies, 69
MiMeDB, 131–132
mineral water, 102
Minnesota: immigrants from Thailand in, 191
Molluscum contagiosum, 48, 50
monads, 12
Montgomery, John, 31*f*
Montreal, Canada, 190
Moraxella, 101
Mossi ethnic group, 187–188
mother-baby dyads, 71
Mother-to-Infant trial, 71–72
MRSA (methicillin-resistant *Staphylococcus aureus*), 49–51, 57–58
mucosal adherence, 167–168
multiple sclerosis (MS), 198–199
Murphy, Mary A., 29
mutualists, 49
Mycobacterium avium, 102
mycophenolic acid, 131
mycorrhizal fungi, 25

N

names of bacteria, 94–95
nanopore sequencing, 37
naphthalene, 165
NASA
Hawaii Space Exploration Analog and Simulation IV, 206–207
Mars500 project, 206
National Institute of Biological Standards and Control (NIBSC), 96
National Institutes of Health (NIH), 186
National Registry for FMTs, 180
National Research Council (NRC), 38
naturalists, early, 11

natural mineral water, 102
Neanderthals, 192
Neisseria cinerea, 9*f*
Neolithic subsistence farmers, 188
nervous system, 121–122
neurotransmitters, 132–133
newborn babies, 64, 66*f*
breech babies, 78
caesarean-born, 72–74
first breath, 65
first encounters with microbes, 64–65, 81–82
first microbes, 65
milk-fed, 69
mother-baby dyads, 71
normal fecal calprotectin, 82
normal flora, 67
survival of, 80–82
transfer of anaerobic bacteria from mother to, 74–75
next-generation sequencing, 36
Nightingale, Florence, 16
NIH Swiss mice, 124–125
Nissle, Alfred, 169
NMRI mice, 124, 129
nomadism, 191
normal flora, 13
normal microbiome, 103–104
Novel Prize, 164
NRC (National Research Council), 38
Nugent's criteria, 158–159
nutrients
dietary, 103
micronutrients, 110
Nuttall, George, 26

O

Obama administration, 37
obesity, 73
observational research, 29
obstetrics, 139

Index 245

ocean environmental research, 31–33
ocean microbiome, 23–24
omnivores, 109, 193–194, 201–202
One Health movement, 25
online stool tests, 87
Open Field Test (OF or OFT), 125, 129
Oscillibacter sp., 105–106
O'Toole, Elizabeth, 70

P

Paleolithic diets, 205
Paneth cells, 80–81
Paraprevotellaceae, 189–190
parasites, 8*f*, 12
PARSIFAL study (Prevention of Allergy—
Risk Factors for Sensitization Related
to Farming and Anthroposophic
Lifestyle), 200
Pasteur, Louis, 12, 17, 22, 26
Pasteur Institute, 164
PASTURE group (Protection
Against Allergy—Study in Rural
Environments), 200
pathogens, 18–19, 80
on skin, 49
in tap water, 102
PATRIC (Pathosystem Resource
Integration Centre) list, 49
Payne, J. F., 62
Pediococcus acidilactici, 100
Penicillium, 100
penis, 143, 147
penis microbiome, 156–157
periodic asthma, 198
petri dishes, 46
Peyer's patches, 80–81
Philadelphia, Pennsylvania, 189
pigment cells, 42
pilosebaceous units, 44
pioneer microbes, 65
pituitary gland, 116, 120, 128–131

placental microbiome, 75–76
plagues, 14–15
plankton, 23–24
plants, 5
points of contact, 57–58
postbiotics, 132, 162, 167
post-puerperal infection, 147–149
prebiotics, 162, 167
pregnancy, 149–150
premature babies, 175–176
Prevoltellaceae, 189–190
Prevotella, 103, 153, 187–188, 190, 191
Price, Philip B., 54–57, 62
Priou, Marie, 166
probiotics, 164, 183
adverse events, 175, 183
for antibiotic-associated
diarrhea, 173–174, 177
capsules, 174
claims about, 170–171
definition of, 161–163
effective, 167–168
evidence for, 172
example microbes, 168–169
first-ever, 166–167
generally recognized as safe (GRAS)
status, 170–171, 174
guidelines for use, 172–174
for irritable bowel syndrome, 174
labeling, 170
market for, 162
metagenomic findings, 176–178
novel, 182
regulation of, 169–171
research findings, 171–173, 174–175,
183
safety of, 174–176
probiotic sepsis, 175–176
Proctor, Lita, 39
Prokaryotes, 23
Prontosil, 149

246 INDEX

Proprionibacterium, 53–54
protists, 23
protozoa, 5, 8*f*, 94
Prozac (fluoxetine), 133
Pseudomonas, 60, 101
Pseudomonas aeruginosa (formerly known as
    Bacillus pyocyaneus), 49, 102
public health, 15–16
Pyrosequencing 454, 35

Q

qualified health claims, 170
Queen Charlotte's Obstetric
    Hospital, 147–148

R

radiotherapy, 181
Ravel, J., 153
Ready to Use Supplementary Food
    (RUSF), 112
red blood cells, 8–9
refeeding formulations, 112
regulation of probiotics, 169–171
research, 208–209
    citizen science, 154–155
    data gathering, 186
    diversity of, 185–186
    double-blind trials, 171–172
    early, 142–143
    environmental, 31–33
    germ-free, 29, 31
    lab mice, 123–127
    low- or no-biomass, 77–80
    metagenomic techniques, 176
    microbiome-gut-brain studies, 116
    microbiome-gut-brain studies in
        mice, 127–130
    microbiome projects, 39
    neonatal, 68–71
    observational, 29
    ocean environmental, 31–33

on probiotics, 171–175
reliability of, 94–98
samples to help standardize results, 96
on vaginal microbiome, 142–143
residents, 49
rewilding, 203–206
rhizosphere, 25
Rhodanobacter, 78–79
Rhodotorula, 48
ribosomal RNA (rRNA), 33
ribosomes, 33
ruminants, 109
Ruminobacter, 191
Ruminococcus, 96
rural areas, 187–188
RV Weatherbird II, 35

S

Saccharomyces, 94
Saccharomyces boulardii, 169, 173
Saccharomyces cerevisiae, 6*f*
safe sex, 4
safety
    generally recognized as safe (GRAS)
        status, 170–171, 174
    of probiotics, 174–176
Sahara, 22
St. Louis, Missouri, 189
salmonella, 93
sand particles, 22
sanitary conditions, 15–16
sanitation, 18–19
saprophytes, 13
Sargasso Sea, 32–35
satiety, 121
SCFAs (short-chain fatty acids), 107, 132,
    136–137
SCID (severe combined immunodeficiency
    disease), 28
Scopulariopsis, 100

SDD (selective decontamination of the digestive tract), 165
sea spray water particles, 22
seborrheic dermatitis, 50
second-generation sequencing, 36
selective decontamination of the digestive tract (SDD), 165
selective serotonin reuptake inhibitors (SSRIs), 133–134
self-infection. *see* autoinfection
Semmelweis, Ignaz Philipp, 139
sepsis, 141, 175–176
SeqCode registry, 95
serotonin, 121, 133–134
severe combined immunodeficiency disease (SCID), 28
sexual infections, 156
sexual intercourse, 4, 155
sexually transmitted diseases (STDs), 152–153
Shattuck, Lemuel, 16
Shigella, 93
Shigella dysenteriae, 34
Shirota, Minoru, 169
short-chain fatty acids (SCFAs), 107, 132, 136–137
shotgun metagenomic sequencing, 34
shotgun sequencing, 36
skin
  as habitat for microbes, 44–46
  structure of, 42–43f, 43
skin cells, 8–9
skin conditions, 61–63
skin flora, 45
  cryptogamic, 61–62
  transients, 55–56
  transplants, 181
skin infections, 50
skin microbiome, 41
  density of variable bacteria in, 45–46
  key transmitters of, 52–54

of newborn babies, 66–67
size of bacterial load on our hands, 55–56
washing and, 54–57
skin pH, 60
skin temperature, 45
small intestine, 90–91, 107
smallpox, 15
smegma, 156
Smith, James, 10–11
soap, 18–19
  antibacterial products, 60
  vs hand sterilizer, 57–61
soil microbiome, 24–25
Sphingomonas, 101
Spirillum, 12–13
Spirochaeteae, 189–190
Spirochaetes, 11
SSRIs (selective serotonin reuptake inhibitors), 134
Staphylococcus, 47–50, 53, 73, 156–157
Staphylococcus aureus, 49–50, 63, 146
  methicillin-resistant (MRSA), 49–51, 57–58
Staphylococcus epidermidis, 46, 50–52, 63, 78–79, 145–146, 156–157
STDs (sexually transmitted diseases), 152–153
Stenotrophomonas, 101
sterile environments
  maintenance of, 27–28
  newborn babies, 75–77
  survival in, 26–27
sterilization
  in childbirth, 139
  hand, 57–61, 139
stomach, 90–91
stool, 91
  fossilized, 192
  non-healthy, 105–106
stool analysis, 87, 90

248 INDEX

stool bacteria, 72, 91, 103
stool microbiomes
  of babies with colic, 83
  diversity in, 186
  of malnourished children, 111–112
  of newborn babies, 72
stool samples, 91–93, 209
Strachan, David P., 199
stratum basale, 42
stratum corneum, 42–43
Streptococcus, 53, 91–93, 145–147, 156–157
Streptococcus agalactiae, 158
Streptococcus faecalis, 70
Streptococcus pyogenes, 49, 147–148
Streptococcus thermophilus, 100
stress response, 115–116, 118, 120,
  128–129
structure/function claims, 170
Subdoligranulum sp., 105–106
Succinovibrionaceae, 189–190
sugar, 103
superorganisms, 210–211
supplements, 112, 182–183
Sweden: neonatal research in, 70–71
Swiss Webster mice, 124, 129
Switzerland, 200
synbiotics, 162
syphilis, 15, 143

T
tap water, 101–102
Teknoscienze, 164
temporal core, 106
terminology, 11–13, 21, 94–95, 210
testicular microbiome, 158
Thailand: immigrants from, 191
Thaumarchaeota, 48
therapies in the pipeline, 181–182
Thucydides, 14–15
Tissier, Henri, 70, 169
toilets, 102–103

transients, 49, 55–56
translational science, 39–40
transplantation. *see also* fecal microbiota
    transplants (FMTs)
  skin microbiome transplants, 181
  vaginal microbiota transplants, 181
Treponema, 191
Treponema succinifaciens, 187–190, 192
Trichomonadidae, 94
Trichomonas vaginalis, 152
Trier Institute of Midwifery, 142
tryptophan, 134
tuberculosis (TB), 143
typhus, 15

U
UK Biobank, 105
ulcerative colitis, 172
United Kingdom
  asthma in, 198–199
  microbiome projects, 39
United States
  Human Microbiome Project
    (HMP), 37–40
  infectious disease in, 202–203
  Obama administration, 37
  probiotic market, 162
  smaller microbiome projects, 39
University of Notre Dame, 29
Unna, Paul Gerson, 61–62
urban areas, 187–188, 193, 195–196
urethra
  female, 157
  male, 157–158
urethral microbiome, 158
urine, 157
US Department of
    Agriculture–recommended
    diet, 100
uterine environment, 77, 79

Index   249

V

vaginal bacillus, 144–145
vaginal bacteria, 71–72, 142–143
vaginal discharge, 144–145
vaginal examination, 139, 140*f*, 149–150
vaginal microbiome(s)
  community state types (CST), 153–154
  CST Group I, 153
  CST Group II, 153
  CST Group III, 153–155
  CST Group IV, 153–155
  CST Group V, 153
  early research on, 142–143
  lifestyle factors, 154–155
  microbes in, 144–145, 145*f*, 147–154
  pH, 153
vaginal microbiota transplants, 181
vaginal smears, 144, 145*f*
vaginosis. *see* bacterial vaginosis (BV)
vagus nerve, 119*f*, 120, 130–131
VANISH taxa (Volatile and/or Associated
    Negatively with Industrialised Societies
    of Humans taxa), 189–190
Vaseline, 141
vegetable growth, 13
vegetables, 103
vegetation, cryptogamic, 13, 18
Veillonella parvula, 47–48
Vetter, David, 28, 30–31, 31*f*, 64
Vibrio, 12–13, 17
Victorians, 22
Vienna General Hospital, 139
virulent streptococci, 145–147
viruses, 7–8, 10*f*
  in gut, 94, 100
  in ocean, 23–24
  size of, 8–9
  in skin, 48

vitamin C, 110–111
vitamin K, 110

W

washing. *see also* handwashing
  effects on skin microbiome, 54–57
water
  bottled, 102
  drinking, 101–102
  tap, 101–102
Welch, William H., 46, 50, 62
Western countries, 186, 198
Western diet, 187
Westernization, 190
Western lifestyle, 202–203
Whipps, J. M., 1
white muscadine, 14
WHO. *see* World Health Organization
whole metagenomic shotgun
    sequencing, 36
Whytt, Robert, 117–120
Wilson, Raphael, 29–30
Woese, Carl R., 32
World Health Organization
    (WHO), 22–23, 54, 85
  definition of probiotics, 161–162
  guidelines for handwashing, 58–59
  guidelines for vaginal examination in
      pregnancy, 149–150
  key health messages, 212
  samples to help standardize research
      results, 96

Y

Yakult, 169
Yanomami tribe, 186, 189–190
yeasts, 6*f*, 6, 12
  example probiotics, 169
  size of, 8–9
yellow fever, 15
yogurt, 164, 166